THE SMART PATIENT'S HEALTHCARE HANDBOOK

A Guide for Taking Control of Your Health

Laura Kuligowska

To Everyone who has been in a doctor's office and thought,
"There must be something else I can do..."

If these worksheets can help you develop more confidence with your doctor, help you create preventative health-management and lifestyle changes, empower you if you are surprised with a frightening diagnosis, or help monitor a loved one through a serious illness, then my dream will be fully realized.

TABLE OF CONTENTS

This book is not intended to diagnose, treat, cure or prevent any disease. The intention is for you to gather information about your own health in one place and use that information in combination with your doctor to make the best decisions to manage your health.

JOIN ME ON YOUTUBE
For
The Smart Patients Healthcare Handbook Video Workshop

This workshop will be my first playlist and a permanent part of my YouTube channel. In the playlist, each section will have its own video and together we will fill in the answers that are unique to you. We will talk about how to use each section to its fullest potential and alternate ways to use the worksheets to suit your unique needs.

INTRODUCTION

For many years, I listened to stories from my nutrition stores' clientele about their on-going frustration with their healthcare. I would listen as they talked about their uncomfortable relationships with their doctors. I saw the fear in their eyes when they confided to me that they had been diagnosed with a serious condition. Amazingly, what I discovered was the reluctance by many to ask their doctors for more information or discuss alternative practices for their illnesses. Of course, this lack of reliable information only escalated their fears and frustrations. I wanted to help my clients, as well as my family and friends, not only in their time of extreme need, but also, I wanted to prevent them from getting to that desperate time in the first place.

I wondered how all these issues could be resolved successfully. Was there something I could do to facilitate a patient's journey through the labyrinth of a confusing and intimidating healthcare system? From those initial thoughts and concerns, **The Smart Patient's Healthcare Handbook was created.**

This interactive handbook is an organizational tool to turn the business of your good health into a corporation where you are the president and your doctor is a very important and *trusted* advisor. By establishing this kind of working relationship with your healthcare providers, you will be treated with more respect, acquire more information, and have comprehensive documentation which will enable you to make better decisions. Ultimately, through your efforts, you will achieve better health.

Throughout my work life, I have created notebooks, workbooks, and presentation books to gather important information. Why not create the same type of tool to gather our health and wellness information? During lunch with some friends, I confessed to them that I was creating *The Smart Patient's Healthcare Handbook*. When one of my dearest friends expressed her wish that she had had a handbook like this during her mother's cancer, I knew I was on the right track. *The Smart Patient's Healthcare Handbook* is available to everyone who needs an easy way to organize and manage one's own health and the health of their family.

TAKING CONTROL

In this new era of the *ten-minute doctor appointment*, we need to be better prepared for each visit to our doctor. Many of us feel we do not have enough time in our appointments with our doctor. The biggest complaint I heard from clients is that when they are with the doctor, they cannot get their questions asked, nor get others answered, because they had felt hurried or they have forgotten their questions altogether.

Maybe you have one of the many healthcare providers where a nurse or physician's assistant gathers most, if not all, of your information. Your doctor then arrives for a short consultation with you, to dole out a prescription, or take a sample of some sort, before racing out of the room and on to the next patient. Because of time constraints, it is difficult for doctors to offer the best choices for you if you do not take a proactive role in your own healthcare.

It is now more important than ever for you to have your questions and concerns at your fingertips to empower you to take a more active role in your own healthcare and to better manage the care of your family.

This handbook can be an-easy-to-use tool that will help you take that more active role. *Remember, not even your own doctor knows as much about your health as you do.*

Even if you are lucky enough to have a healthcare provider who can spend as much time with you at each appointment as necessary now, that may not always be the case. Your healthcare provider can change for any number of reasons, completing this handbook and keeping it up to date, will help you navigate those changes seamlessly. This simple tool will help keep you on top of your current health status and enable you to map out your long-term health program. Changing healthcare providers or plans will be easier if you are in control of your own data.

Concerned doctors want to answer your questions and spend more time with you. They have taken an oath to do everything they can to help you achieve and maintain good health. The better the information you compile for them, the better their diagnosis and treatment will be. This handbook has been designed to give you more control over the time spent with your doctor by giving you the tools to be prepared, to ask the right questions, and to get the care you deserve.

Unfortunately, many doctors today must work within rules set down by insurance companies or government agencies. Insurance companies and the government look at healthcare differently than doctors and patients do. Insurance companies and government bureaucrats require paperwork and cost-containment objectives that may conflict with the amount of time doctors are able to spend at each appointment. The number of patients per doctor alone can diminish time spent per patient. The documentation a doctor must provide to request certain tests, or to refer you to a specialist, also limits the time they can spend with you.

With medical practices seeing more patients in less time, your doctor needs you, the patient, to give them accurate information. It is more important than ever that you have your questions ready and can communicate your current health status clearly, to make the most of your brief meeting. This handbook will help you to be prepared and to plan.

Along with documenting your personal health status, it is important to keep good records on which insurance company or government program currently covers you. Often a change in your healthcare provider may be out of your control. When these changes occur, it will become even more critical for you to be in possession of your own health information.

This handbook provides you with the forms and worksheets necessary to organize your healthcare. With your healthcare information in your control, you will have a complete resource guide to overcome unanticipated changes in your health status, or in your healthcare plan.

This handbook can also be used as a resource to keep you one step ahead of the game by mapping out a strategy for prevention. With so many innovations in healthcare, it can sometimes be dangerous to rely only on your memory when discussing your health history with your doctor. You could miss out on new and innovative treatments that can be provided in the earliest stages of a potentially serious condition by not remembering to mention an illness that runs in your family. You may not be offered an early-detection test that would reveal a hereditary condition that may run in your family only because you neglected to request it from your doctor or from any new doctor that you are assigned.

The Smart Patient's Healthcare Handbook will become a book about your health plan, your health status, and your prevention road map. It can become your voice if your health becomes complicated.

Pencils ready! You are about to create the book of you!

YOUR HEALTH PLAN AND PROVIDERS

This worksheet is your quick-reference about your current health plan provider and all the coverage to which you are entitled. The first worksheet to complete in your handbook will be the *Healthcare Plan and Providers Worksheet*.

Begin by filling in the name of your insurance company, policy number, website address, email and phone number. This information can change annually, so I suggest you write this in pencil.

Healthcare coverage can vary wildly and changes annually so having a place for the details of your current plan for co-pay and such can be placed in the notes section. Place details about how your plan works in that section and again I would recommend using a pencil.

If your healthcare is provided via a government agency or government plan, the name of the information to write on the *Healthcare Plan and Providers Worksheet* may be titled differently than on the worksheet, these titles are a place holder title for your information. Write in those spaces the appropriate information for your plan system and use the notes section to briefly overview how your plan works.

Write in your primary care physician and your preferred pharmacy. You might want to create a location in your smart phone where you store all these contacts for quick access.

Some plans recommend, if possible, for you to use an urgent care center in lieu of an emergency room and give you financial incentive to do so. If you are really ill, your healthcare provider should be able to see you right away. Most doctors have small gaps in their schedule to squeeze in their patient who have urgent needs; that is why sometimes, even when you have an appointment time, you have to wait. More than likely that doctor squeezed in a suddenly ill patient. Which knocks everyone back a bit in line.

You should know the closest urgent care location and phone number. It might also be a good idea to go to the location, that way the first time you go is not when you are in a panic. See how long it takes to get there. Take a minute and put that urgent care information in your smart phone as well.

Dental and vision with employer provided insurance are often covered under different policy numbers. Note the policy number or coverage name in the space provided.

The *Healthcare Plan and Providers Worksheet* has space for dental, vision, chiropractic, psychological, and other health and wellness providers you may frequent. Some insurance companies include coverage for these medical services. If they are covered services, you may want to note that next to the service by writing yes or no.

Take a few moments to review and fill in your *Healthcare Plan and Providers Worksheet* on the following page. As mentioned previously, it may be useful to also create a place in your phone for all your medical contact information.

Healthcare Plan and Providers Worksheet

Healthcare/Insurance provider:_____Policy Number:_____
_____Phone Number:_____
Website:_____Email:_____
Notes: _____
_____
_____
_____

Primary Care Physician:_____Phone Number:_____
Address:_____Email:_____

Preferred Pharmacy Address:_____Phone Number:_____
Back-up Pharmacy Address:_____Phone Number:_____

Closest Urgent Care Facility:_____Phone Number:_____

Closest Hospital Emergency Unit:_____Phone Number:_____

Dental Plan Provider:_____Phone Number:_____
Address:_____Policy No.:_____Email:_____

Optical Plan Provider:_____Phone Number:_____
Address:_____Policy No.:_____Email:_____

Additional Healthcare Contacts

Medical Specialist for: *Chiropractic* Care_____Phone Number:_____
Doctor:_____Covered?_____Address:_____

Medical Specialist for: *Psychological* Care_____Phone Number:_____
Doctor:_____Covered?_____Address:_____

Medical Specialist for:_____Phone Number:_____
Doctor:_____Covered?_____Address:_____

Medical Specialist for:_____Phone Number:_____
Doctor:_____Covered?_____Address:_____

Medical Specialist for:_____Phone Number:_____
Doctor:_____Covered?_____Address:_____

Medical Specialist for:_____Phone Number:_____
Doctor:_____Covered?_____Address:_____

Medical Specialist for:_____ Phone Number:_____
Doctor:_____ Covered?_____ Address:_____

Medical Specialist for:_____ Phone Number:_____
Doctor:_____ Covered?_____ Address:_____

Medical Specialist for:_____ Phone Number:_____
Doctor:_____ Covered?_____ Address:_____

Medical Specialist for:_____ Phone Number:_____
Doctor:_____ Covered?_____ Address:_____

Medical Specialist for:_____ Phone Number:_____
Doctor:_____ Covered?_____ Address:_____

Medical Specialist for:_____ Phone Number:_____
Doctor:_____ Covered?_____ Address:_____

Medical Specialist for:_____ Phone Number:_____
Doctor:_____ Covered?_____ Address:_____

Medical Specialist for:_____ Phone Number:_____
Doctor:_____ Covered?_____ Address:_____

Medical Specialist for:_____ Phone Number:_____
Doctor:_____ Covered?_____ Address:_____

Medical Specialist for:_____ Phone Number:_____
Doctor:_____ Covered?_____ Address:_____

Medical Specialist for:_____ Phone Number:_____
Doctor:_____ Covered?_____ Address:_____

Medical Specialist for:_____ Phone Number:_____
Doctor:_____ Covered?_____ Address:_____

Medical Specialist for:_____ Phone Number:_____
Doctor:_____ Covered?_____ Address:_____

Medical Specialist for:_____ Phone Number:_____
Doctor:_____ Covered?_____ Address:_____

Medical Specialist for:_____ Phone Number:_____
Doctor:_____ Covered?_____ Address:_____

Medical Specialist for:_____ Phone Number:_____
Doctor:_____ Covered?_____ Address:_____

YOUR HEALTH HISTORY

Now that you have a quick reference for your healthcare plan, let's look back and see where you have been.

This brings us to the next worksheet in your handbook, The *Health History Worksheet*. The *Health History Worksheet* gives insight for planning preventative strategies for your health future. It is important to know what conditions and illnesses may be hereditary. Many conditions can be prevented, cured, or controlled if detected early enough.

Many serious illnesses can be detected by genetic testing years before the illnesses would manifest themselves. This information can provide you with the luxury of time. It also allows you to make decisions regarding treatment and lifestyle changes without the pressure and fear that accompanies a sudden serious diagnosis. The more you know about your health history and your immediate family's health history, the better you and your doctor can plot a course of action that maximizes your good health.

When you visit a doctor for the first time, you fill out a *new patient application*. This application asks many questions about your health and the health of your immediate family. I have often wondered if my doctors actually *review* my *new patient application* at each appointment before examining me. The following stories are good examples of why this is a question worth asking.

My grandfather passed from complications associated with diabetes. Some of my grandfather's siblings also had diabetes, as did my maternal great-grandfather. Even though I had noted on my *new patient application* that diabetes runs in my family, my doctor never suggested a blood test to look at my blood sugar levels, nor had he ever asked me any questions that would detect the beginning symptoms of diabetes. This doctor never reviewed with me what symptoms I should consider important and for which I should be on the alert. He never explained *any* prevention strategies against diabetes, like keeping my weight down, exercising, and maintaining my sugar intake in the low to moderate range.

When I first became interested in health and nutrition in my mid-twenties, the possibility that I might contract diabetes became one of my greatest concerns. I asked my doctor to do a blood sugar test. The results indicated that my blood sugar level was on the high side of normal. Fortunately, because of the results of that test, I have made some minor changes in my diet and exercise routine to stay on the safe side of this debilitating disease. The minor lifestyle changes I have made keep my blood sugar in the good range. With even a possible genetic predisposition in this area, I certainly do not want to keep habits that would lay the foundation for future disease.

This is but one example why we, as patients, need to take command of our own health. The possibility exists that my doctor may never have suggested a blood sugar test until I began manifesting obvious symptoms or reached the age when they typically start testing for that. When my blood sugar test had come back on the high side of normal, my doctor said there was *no problem* since it was still in the normal range. *I disagreed.* For me, the high side of normal was too close to diabetes. I could have chosen not to make any lifestyle changes, but knowledge gave me the power to make the changes. I had the information necessary to make an important decision about my health…and all because I had asked *one* question.

My next-door neighbor learned the importance of having accurate medical history information at her fingertips. *Julia's doctor had prescribed a medication for her, however, she happened to be allergic to this medication. Luckily, she reviewed the doctor's illegible prescription notice with the nurse, when she realized it was a medication she could not have, Julia told the nurse to alert the doctor. The doctor then wrote an alternate prescription. Unbelievably, this time it was for another medication to which she was allergic.*

Julia confided to me that she was very disappointed in her doctor because it was obvious that her doctor had not reviewed her chart for possible allergies to medication. In this case, Julia was fortunate. If she had not paid close attention to her prescription, and discussed it with her nurse, the outcome may have had a much different ending. Would you have noticed a life-endangering mistake at the pharmacy? Or even worse, after taking the medication and becoming even more ill? Accurate health history information at your fingertips and asking questions allows you to avoid these types of medical consequences.

The *Health History Worksheet* may be the most detailed worksheet to complete and requires you to talk seriously with your immediate family members about a scary subject: *illness.*

The *Health History Worksheet* moves outward from you and then on to collect as accurate information as possible about your parents, aunts, uncles, grandparents and siblings. You might make a phone call, send a letter, or email explaining what you are doing to gather more family health information. You may have to rely on family members' memories for the health information about any relatives who have passed. It is not necessary to find out all your family health information in one sitting, this is not a one and done workbook. You can gather this information over time as it naturally becomes known. Everyone's relationship to family members is unique I trust you will know the best way to collect any family health information for your *Health History Worksheet.*

If possible when filling in your *Health History Worksheet* try to get as much information about your immediate and late relatives' overall health. You would not want to miss the important health information that no one discussed, such as an Aunt who might have won a private battle with breast cancer, but then later passes from heart disease. The *Health History Worksheet* is a road map for detecting and treating serious illnesses for you. Make it your goal to gather the most accurate information possible. I just caution you to be respectful as illness is a scary and sometimes touchy subject for some, even though it should not be. The more information that is held up to the light, the better it is for everyone in your family. Not just for prevention, but for supporting and helping someone you might find out is struggling.

In this workbook we will look at siblings, parents and grandparents to detect hereditary conditions. It is worth noting, however, that a hereditary condition can show up during any generation. For example, my mother and grandmother do not have breast cancer. That does not preclude me from developing breast cancer. If I were to be diagnosed with breast cancer, I would inform my entire family immediately so that they could be on alert and add breast cancer to the list of conditions for which my children need to watch. My immediate family would also want to add that to their own *Health History Worksheets* and to their children's as well.

There are some hereditary conditions that will become known at birth or in early childhood. Those genetic conditions would appear on your personal *Heath History Worksheet* and possibly on one of your parents or grandparents' worksheets as well.

The easiest part of your *Health History Worksheet* will be the information about your own health. If possible, consult with your parents about any illnesses you had as a child.

You could try and request your medical records from all your former doctors. With the privacy rules healthcare providers must operate by today, it might not be possible to acquire all your past records, or it may be a long and complicated process. Whatever records you can collect provides you with a much clearer picture of your health. *For most of us just having a good general knowledge of our health and an awareness of what to look out for will be good enough.*

Once you have finished your *Health History Worksheet*, it is very simple to keep it up to date. If you become aware of a relative that has contracted an illness that is hereditary, you will want to add that to your worksheet. Then add this condition to the list for discussion at your next doctor appointment. If you were to develop an illness that your family should be made aware, you would want to add that to your worksheet, as well as notify them, so they can be proactive regarding their own health.

After completing your *Health History Worksheet*, you might find that much of the information you jotted down is unnecessary for the purposes of prevention, you now have a record filled with common childhood illness and minor incidents. It is also quite possible that if your family is anything like mine you were able to discover more information than you needed.

Now begins the task of weeding through that information and transferring the most important pieces to your *Health History Summary Log*. At this point you may be thinking, "This is a lot of work." Trust me, the time you spend putting the basics of your healthcare handbook together is mostly spent *here* with your health history. This history lays the foundation for all the remaining steps to take command of your own health. Once you have completed the first few worksheets, it should take only a few minutes before each visit to your doctor to maintain your healthcare handbook.

Health History Worksheet

Name:_____Birth Year:_____Blood Type:_____

Childhood Illnesses:_____
_____
_____

Allergies:_____
_____
_____

Broken Bones:_____
_____
_____

Surgeries:_____
_____
_____

Hospitalizations:_____
_____
_____
_____
_____

Current Illnesses:_____
_____
_____
_____
_____

Chronic Illnesses:_____
_____
_____
_____
_____

(   ):_____
_____
_____
_____
_____

Health History Worksheet – Mother

Name:_____Birth Year:_____Blood Type:_____

Childhood Illnesses:_____
_____
_____

Allergies:_____
_____
_____

Broken Bones:_____
_____
_____

Surgeries:_____
_____
_____

Hospitalizations:_____
_____
_____
_____
_____

Current Illnesses:_____
_____
_____
_____
_____

Chronic Illnesses:_____
_____
_____
_____
_____

(   ):_____
_____
_____
_____
_____

Health History Worksheet –Grandmother (Maternal)

Name:_____Birth Year:_____Blood Type:_____

Allergies:_____
_____

Surgeries:_____
_____
_____

Hospitalizations:_____
_____
_____
_____

Current Illnesses:_____
_____
_____

Chronic Illnesses:_____
_____
_____
_____

Health History Worksheet – Grandfather (Maternal)

Name:_____Birth Year:_____Blood Type:_____

Allergies:_____
_____

Surgeries:_____
_____
_____

Hospitalizations:_____
_____
_____

Current Illnesses:_____
_____
_____

Chronic Illnesses:_____
_____
_____

Health History Worksheet – Father

Name:_____Birth Year:_____Blood Type:_____

Childhood Illnesses:_____
_____
_____

Allergies:_____
_____
_____

Broken Bones:_____
_____
_____

Surgeries:_____
_____
_____

Hospitalizations:_____
_____
_____
_____
_____

Current Illnesses:_____
_____
_____
_____
_____

Chronic Illnesses:_____
_____
_____
_____
_____

(   ):_____
_____
_____
_____
_____

Health History Worksheet –Grandmother (Paternal)

Name:_____Birth Year:_____Blood Type:_____

Allergies:_____
_____

Surgeries:_____
_____
_____

Hospitalizations:_____
_____
_____
_____

Current Illnesses:_____
_____
_____

Chronic Illnesses:_____
_____
_____
_____

Health History Worksheet – Grandfather (Paternal)

Name:_____Birth Year:_____Blood Type:_____

Allergies:_____
_____

Surgeries:_____
_____
_____

Hospitalizations:_____
_____
_____

Current Illnesses:_____
_____
_____

Chronic Illnesses:_____
_____
_____
_____

Health History Worksheet – Sibling/Relative

Name:_____Birth Year:_____Blood Type:_____

Allergies:_____
_____

Surgeries:_____
_____
_____

Hospitalizations:_____
_____
_____
_____

Current Illnesses:_____
_____
_____

Chronic Illnesses:_____
_____
_____
_____

Health History Worksheet – Sibling/Relative

Name:_____Birth Year:_____Blood Type:_____

Allergies:_____
_____

Surgeries:_____
_____
_____

Hospitalizations:_____
_____
_____
_____

Current Illnesses:_____
_____
_____

Chronic Illnesses:_____
_____
_____

Health History Worksheet – Sibling/Relative

Name:_____Birth Year:_____Blood Type:_____

Allergies:_____
_____

Surgeries:_____
_____
_____

Hospitalizations:_____
_____
_____
_____

Current Illnesses:_____
_____
_____

Chronic Illnesses:_____
_____
_____
_____

Health History Worksheet – Sibling/Relative

Name:_____Birth Year:_____Blood Type:_____

Allergies:_____
_____

Surgeries:_____
_____
_____

Hospitalizations:_____
_____
_____

Current Illnesses:_____
_____
_____

Chronic Illnesses:_____
_____
_____
_____

Health History Worksheet –Sibling/Relative

Name:_____Birth Year:_____Blood Type:_____

Allergies:_____
_____

Surgeries:_____
_____
_____

Hospitalizations:_____
_____
_____
_____

Current Illnesses:_____
_____
_____
_____

Chronic Illnesses:_____
_____
_____
_____

Health History Worksheet – Sibling/Relative

Name:_____Birth Year:_____Blood Type:_____

Allergies:_____
_____

Surgeries:_____
_____
_____

Hospitalizations:_____
_____
_____
_____

Current Illnesses:_____
_____
_____

Chronic Illnesses:_____
_____
_____
_____

Health History Worksheet –Sibling/Relative

Name:_____Birth Year:_____Blood Type:_____

Allergies:_____
_____

Surgeries:_____
_____
_____

Hospitalizations:_____
_____
_____
_____

Current Illnesses:_____
_____
_____

Chronic Illnesses:_____
_____
_____
_____

Health History Worksheet – Sibling/Relative

Name:_____Birth Year:_____Blood Type:_____

Allergies:_____
_____

Surgeries:_____
_____
_____

Hospitalizations:_____
_____
_____

Current Illnesses:_____
_____
_____

Chronic Illnesses:_____
_____
_____
_____

NOTES:

HEALTH HISTORY SUMMARY LOG

The *Health History Summary Log* is the next step in the organization of your health. In this log, you will jot down *only* the conditions that could have an impact on you in the future and that you should be monitoring. Review your *Health History Worksheets* and transfer the information about your hereditary conditions to your summary log. The *Health History Summary Log* can be reviewed before each doctor's appointment. Reviewing this log will help you formulate proactive questions for your doctor. Together you can decide what, if any, actions should be taken based on your detailed family history.

If you are not sure which conditions are hereditary, take your *Health History Worksheet* with you on your next office visit and review it with your doctor, nurse, or physician's assistant. Circle the conditions on your *Health History Worksheet* that should be transferred to your *Health History Summary Log* for future review. You might want to take this opportunity to have a conversation with your doctor about prevention strategies.

If your next office visit is far off in the future. You can do some research on the internet. Search "Is XYZ a hereditary condition?" If you determine that you do indeed have the possibility of contracting a hereditary illness or condition in the future, you would want to confirm with your doctor that the condition is indeed hereditary at your next visit. Then discuss any of the early warning signs to look out for and any some prevention strategies you can employ. You could also continue your research online to see what lifestyle changes you might make now to prolong your good health.

If an illness runs in your family, it is not certain that you will also contract that illness. It doesn't hurt to have knowledge and the opportunity to make change *now* in the unlikely event you should inherit that illness too. *Making changes for better health are never bad changes to make.*

Health History Summary Log

A summary of all conditions that should be monitored

Using the Health History Worksheets as a guide, enter the illnesses and allergies in your family history including your own, that should be monitored. This page should be reviewed in the waiting room before each appointment. Reviewing your log before appointments can help you to formulate proactive questions for your doctor.

Relation	Illness/Allergy	When Contracted	Current Status	My Plan

WHAT TEST AT WHAT AGE LOG

It would be impossible for anyone to anticipate every test you would ever need to protect you from every possible condition. The *What Tests At What Age Log* includes some of the tests that are generally recommended. You and your doctor will add others that are specific for your situation to maintain your good health. As new medical testing information becomes available, you may want to add those new tests onto your log in the appropriate age category. With the many health segments on the news and health shows on television, radio and the internet, you may also hear of a test that is appropriate for future consideration to put on your test log.

Both you and your doctor may use the *What Tests At What Age Log* as a quick reference guide. In combination with your *Health History Worksheet*, both you and your doctor can review the test log and change what is appropriate to your health history, current vital statistics, and any on-going conditions.

As we age, we become more susceptible to certain conditions. While it is impossible to foresee every disease, there are a few that can be detected early if you are attentive to the signs. With this handbook, you will be more aware, and thus able to make better decisions about your health.

Following are just a few of the types of conditions that will appear on your *What Tests At What Age Log*, and why. You and your doctor will add more as you become more proactive with your prevention program.

Blood Pressure Test
Blood pressure tracking is an important part of the *Vital Statistics Tracking Charts*. High Blood Pressure is also known as *the silent killer*, because often you can feel fine until it becomes critical. High blood pressure has a tendency to run in families, with men seeing higher pressures in their mid-thirties and women after menopause. African-Americans have a higher occurrence of high blood pressure that comes on earlier in life and can be more severe. If you have a family history of hypertension, or are African-American, be vigilant with your blood pressure tracking chart, and discuss any changes with your doctor, even if you feel great. If you are over thirty-five at high risk and not seeing your doctor annually, please, get your blood pressure checked. Invest in a blood pressure testing kit or visit the blood pressure kiosk at your local pharmacy.

Cholesterol Test
Some doctors consider high cholesterol levels as an indicator of future problems of the heart and arteries. Recent research regarding Cholesterol is changing our view of Cholesterol and some research has found that individuals with higher levels show no signs of heart and artery disease. For Cholesterol testing you may want to work closely with your doctor based on your personal history to develop a useful testing schedule.

Blood Sugar Test
Diabetes comes in two forms, Type I and Type II. Both types of Diabetes are very serious conditions. More than half of diabetics also have high blood pressure. Individuals with diabetes have more than double the risk of stroke, and heart and artery diseases. Diabetes is the leading cause of end-stage kidney disease and adult blindness. More than fifty percent of limb amputations in the U.S. are in diabetics. If you have a close relative with diabetes you are more likely to develop the disease.

Type II typically develops in individuals over the age of 40. Diabetes threatens not only the length of your life, but also, it threatens the quality of your life. Work with your doctor to start blood sugar testing by at least age 45 to have a *fasting plasma glucose test* and create a future testing schedule with your doctor. If you have risk factors such as a parent, grandparent or siblings with diabetes, you should be tested at a younger age.

Heart Disease Screening

Heart disease can affect anyone. Even individuals with no family history of heart disease should start talking with their doctor about their heart health in their forties. If heart disease runs in your family, you and your doctor may want to have these tests done at an earlier age; or begin watching your *Vital Statistics Tracking Charts* with a more critical eye.

Bone Density Test

Osteoporosis is considered by many a problem only for postmenopausal women. The loss of bone density, however, can occur before menopause. Men are not immune from a loss in bone density. Women may want to ask for a bone density test at the same time they have their baseline breast cancer test, around age 35. Men may want to ask for a bone density check in their mid to late 40s. If osteoporosis runs in your family, it would be wise to have a bone density test about five years earlier.

Cancer Screening

Unfortunately, there are far too many types of cancer, it would be impossible to set up a preventative testing schedule for each one. For the more common cancers, such as breast cancer, colon cancer and skin cancer, tests are now routinely recommended once you hit the age at which they typically appear.

Women should have a PAP test performed by the age of 18, or when they become sexually active, whichever is earlier. If you have a family history of reproductive system cancer, discuss your history with your doctor at every one of your appointments.

Around age 35, women should be discussing a more rigorous breast cancer testing schedule with their doctors. If any of your family members have had breast cancer, discuss a breast cancer testing schedule for early detection before the age of 35 and speak with your doctor about the latest testing procedures at each of your checkups.

Colon and rectal cancer are the most common cancers, most often detected after the age of fifty. Colon and rectal cancers can occur in people at earlier ages. First-degree relatives of a person with colon or rectal cancer are at a higher risk. Individuals who have ulcerative colitis or familial polyposis have an increased risk, as well. Discuss testing for colon and rectal cancers with your doctor, especially if you are in a high-risk group and create a testing schedule to fit your unique situation.

More than half of the men between the ages of 60 and 70, and close to 90% of the men over 70, have symptoms of BPH Benign Prostate Hyperplasia. Men should be tested at the latest by age 55, earlier if you have an increased risk due to family history.

Skin cancer will occur in up to 50% of the population who live to the age of 65. Most of these cancers occur after the age of 50. The greatest risk is to those with fair skin, those who freckle easily, or have light hair and eyes. Most skin cancers begin on the surface of the skin and are easily detected during a thorough skin examination. A monthly self-examination of the skin is recommended for those with the higher risk factors listed above. Skin cancer may run in families, so find out during your Health History fact gathering if any of your relatives have had it. If you find skin cancer in your family history, or have any of the risk factors listed, discuss a skin examination schedule, or a mole mapping with your doctor. A skin examination can easily be worked into your annual checkup.

Lung cancer testing is a *must* for those who choose to use any type of tobacco products. Most lung cancers have a direct relation to tobacco use. Cigarette smokers have a slightly higher risk than cigar or pipe smokers do. Other risk factors would be exposure to asbestos, pollution, radon, and tuberculosis. If you have any of these risk factors, discuss testing schedule with your doctor.

If a type of cancer not mentioned here shows up on your *Health History Worksheet*, discuss a testing schedule with your doctor and add it to the *What Tests At What Age Log* for future use. It is important to be aware of the risk factors so that you can protect yourself. Set up a proper screening schedule with your doctor and avoid bad habits that add to your risk factors.

The tests on your *What Tests At What Age Log* are not the only tests that you may need. The tests listed may not cover hereditary diseases that run in your family and have *early detection testing* already available. You and your doctor should add those tests and others to your list specific to your unique prevention and detection plan. Once those tests are added to your log, it will be easy to remember to request those tests in a timely manner.

As I mentioned earlier, it would be impossible to make a note of every test available. This is just a start. Create a testing program that works with your overall prevention program.

What Tests At What Age Log

Twenties

Female Reproductive System Exam/Pap (Age 18 or when sexually active, then every 3-5 years if normal)
My Results and Plan:_____

Blood Pressure Test (Each Doctor visit)
My Results and Plan:_____

Overall Cholesterol (Age 20 then every 5 years if normal)
My Results and Plan:_____

Blood Sugar Test if you have risk factors, such as family history of Diabetes, High Blood Pressure, Overweight (BMI over 25)
My Results and Plan:_____

Sexually Transmitted Diseases (If you are sexually active) some STDs have no symptoms until it is too late to correct for loss of fertility.
My Results and Plan:_____

Eye Exam once at least in your twenties. Every other year if you need corrective lens.
My Results and Plan:_____

Dental Exam once a year minimum, better to schedule a dental cleaning with exam every six months.
My Plan:_____

Weight. Determine a health weight for your good health and make a proactive plan to maintain your weight by planning healthy eating and moderate exercise.
My Plan:_____
_____
_____

Tests - you and your Doctor add for your personal healthcare needs

Test:_____Testing Schedule:_____
My Results and Plan:_____

Test:_____Testing Schedule:_____
My Results and Plan:_____

Test:_____Testing Schedule:_____
My Results and Plan:_____

Test:_____Testing Schedule:_____
My Results and Plan:_____

Test:_____Testing Schedule:_____
My Results and Plan:_____

*** There is additional space to place testing specific to your unique needs – skip ahead 8 pages ***

What Tests At What Age Log

Thirties

Female Reproductive System Exam/Pap/Breast (Every 3-5 years if normal)
My Results and Plan:_____
Testing Schedule and Type of Screening for Breast Cancer: _____

Blood Pressure Test – (Each Doctor Visit)
My Results and Plan:_____

Overall Cholesterol (Every 5 years if normal)
My Results and Plan:_____

Blood Sugar Test if you have risk factors, such as family history of Diabetes, High Blood Pressure, Overweight (BMI over 25)
My Results and Plan:_____

Sexually Transmitted Diseases (If you are sexually active)
My Results and Plan:_____

Eye Exam once at least in your thirties. Every other year if you need corrective lens.
My Results and Plan:_____

Dental Exam once a year minimum, better to schedule a dental cleaning with exam every six months
My Plan:_____

Weight. Determine a health weight for your good health and make a proactive plan to maintain your weight by planning healthy eating and moderate exercise.
My Plan:_____
_____
_____

Tests - you and your Doctor add for your personal healthcare needs

Test: *Baseline Bone Density for Women* Testing Schedule:_____
My Results and Plan:_____

Test:_____Testing Schedule:_____
My Results and Plan:_____

Test:_____Testing Schedule:_____
My Results and Plan:_____

Test:_____Testing Schedule:_____
My Results and Plan:_____

Test:_____Testing Schedule:_____
My Results and Plan:_____
There is additional space to place testing specific to your unique needs – skip ahead 7 pages

What Tests At What Age Log

Forties

Female Reproductive System Exam/Pap/Breast (Every 3-5 years if normal)
My Results and Plan:_____
Testing Schedule and Type of Screening for Breast Cancer: _____

Blood Pressure Test – (Each Doctor Visit)
My Results and Plan:_____

Overall Cholesterol (Every 5 years if normal)
My Results and Plan:_____

Blood Sugar Test (Regardless of risk factors)
My Results and Plan:_____

Sexually Transmitted Diseases (If you are sexually active)
My Results and Plan:_____

Eye Exam once at least in your forties. Every other year if you need corrective lens.
My Results and Plan:_____

Dental Exam every six months schedule a dental cleaning with exam.
My Plan:_____

Weight. Determine a health weight for your good health and make a proactive plan to maintain your weight by planning healthy eating and moderate exercise.
My Plan:_____
_____
_____

Tests - you and your Doctor add for your personal healthcare needs

Test: _Male Reproductive Exam PSA mid-forties if at high risk of Prostate Cancer_ Testing Schedule:_____
My Results and Plan:_____

Test: _Bone Density Men, Women if not done in thirties_. Testing Schedule:_____
My Results and Plan:_____

Test: _Develop Heart Disease Screening with Doctor_ Testing Schedule:_____
My Results and Plan:_____

Test: _Colon Cancer Screening for those at high risk_ Testing Schedule:_____
My Results and Plan:_____

Test:_____Testing Schedule:_____
My Results and Plan:_____

There is additional space to place testing specific to your unique needs – skip ahead 6 pages

What Tests At What Age Log

Fifties

Female Reproductive System Exam/Pap/Breast (Every 3-5 years if normal)
My Results and Plan:_____
Testing Schedule and Type of Screening for Breast Cancer: _____

Blood Pressure Test – (Each Doctor Visit)
My Results and Plan:_____

Overall Cholesterol (Every 5 years if normal)
My Results and Plan:_____

Blood Sugar Test in accordance with Doctor suggested schedule:
My Results and Plan:_____

Sexually Transmitted Diseases (If you are sexually active)
My Results and Plan:_____

Eye Exam every other year if you need corrective lens.
My Results and Plan:_____

Dental Exam every six months schedule a dental cleaning with exam.
My Plan:_____

Weight. Determine a health weight for your good health and make a proactive plan to maintain your weight by planning healthy eating and moderate exercise.
My Plan:_____
_____
_____

Tests - you and your Doctor add for your personal healthcare needs

Test: *Male Reproductive Exam PSA* Testing Schedule:_____
My Results and Plan:_____

Test: *Heart Disease in accordance with Doctor suggested Testing Schedule*:_____
My Results and Plan:_____

Test: *Colon Cancer Screening, FOBT, FS or Colonoscopy* Testing Schedule:_____
My Results and Plan:_____

Test:_____Testing Schedule:_____
My Results and Plan:_____

Test:_____Testing Schedule:_____
My Results and Plan:_____

There is additional space to place testing specific to your unique needs – skip ahead 5 pages

What Tests At What Age Log

Sixties

Female & Male Reproductive System Exams, with a focus on Screening for Cancer:
My Results and Plan:_____

Blood Pressure Test – (Each Doctor Visit)
My Results and Plan:_____

Overall Cholesterol (Every 5 years if normal)
My Results and Plan:_____

Blood Sugar Test in accordance with Doctor suggested schedule:
My Results and Plan:_____

Sexually Transmitted Diseases (If you are sexually active)
My Results and Plan:_____

Eye Exam every other year if you need corrective lens.
My Results and Plan:_____

Dental Exam every six months schedule a dental cleaning with exam.
My Plan:_____

Weight. Determine a health weight for your good health and make a proactive plan to maintain your weight by planning healthy eating and moderate exercise.
My Plan:_____
_____
_____

Tests - you and your Doctor add for your personal healthcare needs

Test: *Heart Disease in accordance with Doctor suggested* Testing Schedule:_____
My Results and Plan:_____

Test: *Colon Cancer Screening, FOBT, FS or Colonoscopy* Testing Schedule:_____
My Results and Plan:_____

Test:_____Testing Schedule:_____
My Results and Plan:_____

Test:_____Testing Schedule:_____
My Results and Plan:_____

Test:_____Testing Schedule:_____
My Results and Plan:_____

There is additional space to place testing specific to your unique needs – skip ahead 4 pages

What Tests At What Age Log

Seventies

Female & Male Reproductive System Exams, with a focus on Screening for Cancer.
My Results and Plan:_____

Blood Pressure Test – (Each Doctor Visit)
My Results and Plan:_____

Overall Cholesterol (Every 5 years if normal)
My Results and Plan:_____

Blood Sugar Test in accordance with Doctor suggested schedule:
My Results and Plan:_____

Sexually Transmitted Diseases (If you are sexually active)
My Results and Plan:_____

Eye Exam every other year if you need corrective lens.
My Results and Plan:_____

Dental Exam every six months schedule a dental cleaning with exam.
My Plan:_____

Weight. Determine a health weight for your good health and make a proactive plan to maintain your weight by planning healthy eating and moderate exercise.
My Plan:_____
_____
_____

Tests - you and your Doctor add for your personal healthcare needs

Test: *Heart Disease in accordance with Doctor suggested* Testing Schedule:_____
My Results and Plan:_____

Test: *Colon Cancer Screening, FOBT, FS or Colonoscopy* Testing Schedule:_____
My Results and Plan:_____

Test:_____Testing Schedule:_____
My Results and Plan:_____

Test:_____Testing Schedule:_____
My Results and Plan:_____

Test:_____Testing Schedule:_____
My Results and Plan:_____

There is additional space to place testing specific to your unique needs – skip ahead 3 pages

What Tests At What Age Log

Eighties

Female & Male Reproductive System Exams, with a focus on Screening for Cancer.
My Results and Plan:_____

Blood Pressure Test – (Each Doctor Visit)
My Results and Plan:_____

Overall Cholesterol (Every 5 years if normal)
My Results and Plan:_____

Blood Sugar Test in accordance with Doctor suggested schedule:
My Results and Plan:_____

Sexually Transmitted Diseases (If you are sexually active)
My Results and Plan:_____

Eye Exam every other year if you need corrective lens.
My Results and Plan:_____

Dental Exam every six months schedule a dental cleaning with exam.
My Plan:_____

Weight. Determine a health weight for your good health and make a proactive plan to maintain your weight by planning healthy eating and moderate exercise.
My Plan:_____
_____
_____

Tests - you and your Doctor add for your personal healthcare needs

Test: _Heart Disease in accordance with Doctor suggested_ Testing Schedule:_____
My Results and Plan:_____

Test: _Colon Cancer Screening, FOBT, FS or Colonoscopy_ Testing Schedule:_____
My Results and Plan:_____

Test:_____Testing Schedule:_____
My Results and Plan:_____

Test:_____Testing Schedule:_____
My Results and Plan:_____

Test:_____Testing Schedule:_____
My Results and Plan:_____

There is additional space to place testing specific to your unique needs – skip ahead 2 pages

What Tests At What Age Log

Nineties and Beyond

Female & Male Reproductive System Exams, with a focus on Screening for Cancer.
My Results and Plan:_____

Blood Pressure Test – (Each Doctor Visit)
My Results and Plan:_____

Overall Cholesterol (Every 5 years if normal).
My Results and Plan:_____

Blood Sugar Test in accordance with Doctor suggested schedule:
My Results and Plan:_____

Sexually Transmitted Diseases (If you are sexually active)
My Results and Plan:_____

Eye Exam every other year if you need corrective lens.
My Results and Plan:_____

Dental Exam every six months schedule a dental cleaning with exam.
My Plan:_____

Weight. Determine a health weight for your good health and make a proactive plan to maintain your weight by planning healthy eating and moderate exercise.
My Plan:_____
_____
_____

Tests - you and your Doctor add for your personal healthcare needs

Test: _Heart Disease in accordance with Doctor suggested_ Testing Schedule:_____
My Results and Plan:_____

Test: _Colon Cancer Screening, FOBT, FS or Colonoscopy_ Testing Schedule:_____
My Results and Plan:_____

Test:_____Testing Schedule:_____
My Results and Plan:_____

Test:_____Testing Schedule:_____
My Results and Plan:_____

Test:_____Testing Schedule:_____
My Results and Plan:_____

There is additional space to place testing specific to your unique needs – skip ahead next page

Tests for My Good Health

Specific Testing and Tracking for my unique needs not listed in age logs

Place tests and testing schedules that you want to track to maintain your good health that may not be tested for or tracked in a general checkup. Also tests that are important for preventative planning. Any testing and testing schedule that you want to include as a reminder to request the tests, just in case they are not offered as part of a typical exam.

Test:_____Testing Schedule:_____
My Results and Plan:_____

Test:_____Testing Schedule:_____
My Results and Plan:_____

Test:_____Testing Schedule:_____
My Results and Plan:_____

Test:_____Testing Schedule:_____
My Results and Plan:_____

Test:_____Testing Schedule:_____
My Results and Plan:_____

Test:_____Testing Schedule:_____
My Results and Plan:_____

Test:_____Testing Schedule:_____
My Results and Plan:_____

Test:_____Testing Schedule:_____
My Results and Plan:_____

Test:_____Testing Schedule:_____
My Results and Plan:_____

Test:_____Testing Schedule:_____
My Results and Plan:_____

Test:_____Testing Schedule:_____
My Results and Plan:_____

Test:_____Testing Schedule:_____
My Results and Plan:_____

Test:_____Testing Schedule:_____
My Results and Plan:_____

Test:_____Testing Schedule:_____
My Results and Plan:_____

Tests for My Good Health

Specific Testing and Tracking for my unique needs not listed in age logs

Test:_____Testing Schedule:_____
My Results and Plan:_____

Test:_____Testing Schedule:_____
My Results and Plan:_____

Test:_____Testing Schedule:_____
My Results and Plan:_____

Test:_____Testing Schedule:_____
My Results and Plan:_____

Test:_____Testing Schedule:_____
My Results and Plan:_____

Test:_____Testing Schedule:_____
My Results and Plan:_____

Test:_____Testing Schedule:_____
My Results and Plan:_____

Test:_____Testing Schedule:_____
My Results and Plan:_____

Test:_____Testing Schedule:_____
My Results and Plan:_____

Test:_____Testing Schedule:_____
My Results and Plan:_____

Test:_____Testing Schedule:_____
My Results and Plan:_____

Test:_____Testing Schedule:_____
My Results and Plan:_____

Test:_____Testing Schedule:_____
My Results and Plan:_____

Test:_____Testing Schedule:_____
My Results and Plan:_____

Test:_____Testing Schedule:_____
My Results and Plan:_____

NOTES:

IMMUNIZATION LOG

The *Immunization Log* plays a minor role in our adult lives. Unless you are a world traveler, visiting exotic locales that require medical protection from exotic diseases, you have probably had the basic immunizations already.

Your standard immunizations were most likely given to you during childhood. If you know the dates, or even the year, enter them on the log. If you had any side effects to any of those immunizations, log them as well. *In my log I just wrote, standard childhood immunizations given after 1962 in USA. Then added the several tetanus booster shots I've been given over the years.*

There are some immunizations that need refreshing at regular intervals. Review your Immunization Log with your doctor and proceed as needed for your personal health goals.

If you work in childcare or healthcare just like a *world traveler*, you may want to keep your immunizations up to date. In your profession you are exposed to bacteria and viruses. You are at a higher risk of contracting infections than those who do not work in these fields.

Immunization Log

Standard Immunizations *(many of these listed are given before age two)*

Date:_____HB (Hepatitis B)
Date:_____Rotavirus
Date:_____DTaP (Diphtheria, Tetanus & Acellular Pertussis)
Date:_____Hib (Heamophilus Influenzae type b)
Date:_____PCV13 (Pneumococcal Conjugate)
Date:_____IPV (Inactivated Poliovirus)
Date:_____IIV;LAIV (Influenza)
Date:_____MMR (Measles, Mumps & Rubella)
Date:_____Varicella (Chicken Pox/Shingles)
Date:_____HA (Hepatitis A)
Date:_____MenB (Meningococcal type B)
Received all standard immunizations given in _____ year of your birth
Yes:_____No:_____I Don't Know:_____
Personal Notes:_____
_____

Immunizations For Adults To Consider *(work with your doctor to complete this list)*

Date:_____Tetanus/Diphtheria suggested every 10 years as it fades over time
This is routinely given if you have an accident, for example I was given one when I broke my shoulder.
Date:_____HB (Hepatitis B) if not previously immunized, as it is easy to catch
Also known as the "silent epidemic", in the US this has been a routine inoculation since 1991
Date:_____Varicella (Chicken Pox/Shingles)
The CDC claims that this can minimize the chance of the virus "waking up" by boosting your immunity
Date:_____MMR (Measles, Mumps, Rubella) if you have not been infected or immunized
In the US this has been a required inoculation since 1989 due to severe outbreaks at that time.
Date:_____Influenza (Flu) recommended by the CDC for over 50 or in high risk group
Date:_____Pneumococcal (Pneumonia) recommended by the CDC for over 65
High Risk Group: Adults with or living with someone who has cancer, heart, lung or liver diseases, diabetes, weak immunity, etcetera
Date;_____HA (Hepatitis A) recommended by CDC for childcare workers
An extra inoculation for childcare workers to add to the list above, because you are special, in the best way possible.

Log for Immunization you may have received – not listed above

Date:_____Immunization:_____
Date:_____Immunization:_____
Date:_____Immunization:_____
Date:_____Immunization:_____
Date:_____Immunization:_____
Date:_____Immunization:_____
Date:_____Immunization:_____
Date:_____Immunization:_____
Date:_____Immunization:_____
Date:_____Immunization:_____
Date:_____Immunization:_____
Date:_____Immunization:_____
Date:_____Immunization:_____

World Travelers Immunization Record

A handy place to keep track

Some immunizations duplicated from previous list, note the date from previous log to avoid duplication

Date:_____Tetanus/Diphtheria
Date:_____HB (Hepatitis B)
Date:_____HA (Hepatitis A)
Date:_____MMR (Measles, Mumps & Rubella)
Date:_____Polio Booster
Date:_____Yellow Fever
Date:_____Immunization:_____
Date:_____Immunization:_____
Date:_____Immunization:_____
Date:_____Immunization:_____
Date:_____Immunization:_____
Date:_____Immunization:_____
Date:_____Immunization:_____
Date:_____Immunization:_____
Date:_____Immunization:_____
Date:_____Immunization:_____
Date:_____Immunization:_____
Date:_____Immunization:_____
Date:_____Immunization:_____
Date:_____Immunization:_____
Date:_____Immunization:_____
Date:_____Immunization:_____
Date:_____Immunization:_____
Date:_____Immunization:_____
Date:_____Immunization:_____
Date:_____Immunization:_____
Date:_____Immunization:_____
Date:_____Immunization:_____
Date:_____Immunization:_____
Date:_____Immunization:_____
Date:_____Immunization:_____
Date:_____Immunization:_____
Date:_____Immunization:_____
Date:_____Immunization:_____
Date:_____Immunization:_____
Date:_____Immunization:_____
Date:_____Immunization:_____
Date:_____Immunization:_____
Date:_____Immunization:_____

PRESCRIPTION LOG

The *Prescription Log* can be an important tool for gaining and maintaining your good health. Not only can you keep track of prescription drugs you are prescribed or are currently taking, you can also record vitamins, herbs and other remedies about which your doctor should be informed.

You may have a reoccurring condition that requires on-going medication. By writing notes in the side effects and results section, you and your doctor can make decisions about continued use of a prescribed medication.

Your *Prescription Log* should be copied and given to your caregiver if you are ever seriously ill. Your caregiver can then use it to administer your medications, vitamins and herbs. They can also monitor you for any side-effects you experience that you may not notice yourself.

Many people are taking vitamins, herbs, enzymes, homeopathic remedies and other supplements. I recommend you make a note of these types of supplements as if they were medications. Your doctor needs complete information in order to make any diagnosis as accurate as possible. Some vitamins taken in high dosages can cause illness symptoms. Some herbs can cause allergic reactions. In order to rule out these symptoms while making a diagnosis, your doctor must know exactly what you are taking, especially if a symptom is occurring after a new supplement is added to your prevention program.

Many doctors are very knowledgeable about vitamin supplements and can help you incorporate them into your prevention program.

In your handbook, there are several pages of blank *Prescription Logs* for your convenience. You can use one page for medications, and one page for vitamins, etc. Another way to use your *Prescription Log* is to circle the P for prescription, V for vitamin, H for herb, A for amino acid, E for enzyme and HO for homeopathic remedy, in the upper right-hand corner of each block. Finally, you can use a highlighter pen and color code medications in one color, and vitamin supplements in another. Once you decide how to organize your *Prescription Log*, stay consistent with that method to make finding information easier as you continue to monitor your vital health data.

With your groundwork now completed, you are ready for your first office visit. From now on it should only take a few minutes before and after each doctor appointment to keep your handbook in smooth running order.

Prescription Log

Medication:_____ For:_____ P V H A E HO

Dosage Info:_____ Side Effects:_____

_____

Start Date:_____ Stop Date:_____

Result?_____

Medication:_____ For:_____ P V H A E HO

Dosage Info:_____ Side Effects:_____

_____

Start Date:_____ Stop Date:_____

Result?_____

Medication:_____ For:_____ P V H A E HO

Dosage Info:_____ Side Effects:_____

_____

Start Date:_____ Stop Date:_____

Result?_____

Medication:_____ For:_____ P V H A E HO

Dosage Info:_____ Side Effects:_____

_____

Start Date:_____ Stop Date:_____

Result?_____

Medication:_____ For:_____ P V H A E HO

Dosage Info:_____ Side Effects:_____

_____

Start Date:_____ Stop Date:_____

Result?_____

P=Prescription, V=Vitamin, H=Herb, A=Amino Acid, E=Enzyme, HO=Homeopathic Remedy

Prescription Log

Medication:_____ For:_____ P V H A E HO

Dosage Info:_____ Side Effects:_____

_____

Start Date:_____ Stop Date:_____

Result?_____

Medication:_____ For:_____ P V H A E HO

Dosage Info:_____ Side Effects:_____

_____

Start Date:_____ Stop Date:_____

Result?_____

Medication:_____ For:_____ P V H A E HO

Dosage Info:_____ Side Effects:_____

_____

Start Date:_____ Stop Date:_____

Result?_____

Medication:_____ For:_____ P V H A E HO

Dosage Info:_____ Side Effects:_____

_____

Start Date:_____ Stop Date:_____

Result?_____

Medication:_____ For:_____ P V H A E HO

Dosage Info:_____ Side Effects:_____

_____

Start Date:_____ Stop Date:_____

Result?_____

P=Prescription, V=Vitamin, H=Herb, A=Amino Acid, E=Enzyme, HO=Homeopathic Remedy

Prescription Log

Medication:_____ For:_____ P V H A E HO

Dosage Info:_____ Side Effects:_____

_____

Start Date:_____ Stop Date:_____

Result?_____

Medication:_____ For:_____ P V H A E HO

Dosage Info:_____ Side Effects:_____

_____

Start Date:_____ Stop Date:_____

Result?_____

Medication:_____ For:_____ P V H A E HO

Dosage Info:_____ Side Effects:_____

_____

Start Date:_____ Stop Date:_____

Result?_____

Medication:_____ For:_____ P V H A E HO

Dosage Info:_____ Side Effects:_____

_____

Start Date:_____ Stop Date:_____

Result?_____

Medication:_____ For:_____ P V H A E HO

Dosage Info:_____ Side Effects:_____

_____

Start Date:_____ Stop Date:_____

Result?_____

P=Prescription, V=Vitamin, H=Herb, A=Amino Acid, E=Enzyme, HO=Homeopathic Remedy

Prescription Log

Prescription Log

Medication:_____ For:_____ P V H A E HO

Dosage Info:_____ Side Effects:_____

_____

Start Date:_____ Stop Date:_____

Result?_____

Medication:_____ For:_____ P V H A E HO

Dosage Info:_____ Side Effects:_____

_____

Start Date:_____ Stop Date:_____

Result?_____

Medication:_____ For:_____ P V H A E HO

Dosage Info:_____ Side Effects:_____

_____

Start Date:_____ Stop Date:_____

Result?_____

Medication:_____ For:_____ P V H A E HO

Dosage Info:_____ Side Effects:_____

_____

Start Date:_____ Stop Date:_____

Result?_____

Medication:_____ For:_____ P V H A E HO

Dosage Info:_____ Side Effects:_____

_____

Start Date:_____ Stop Date:_____

Result?_____

P=Prescription, V=Vitamin, H=Herb, A=Amino Acid, E=Enzyme, HO=Homeopathic Remedy

Prescription Log

Medication:_____For:_____ | P V H A E HO |

Dosage Info:_____Side Effects:_____

_____

Start Date:_____Stop Date:_____

Result?_____

Medication:_____For:_____ | P V H A E HO |

Dosage Info:_____Side Effects:_____

_____

Start Date:_____Stop Date:_____

Result?_____

Medication:_____For:_____ | P V H A E HO |

Dosage Info:_____Side Effects:_____

_____

Start Date:_____Stop Date:_____

Result?_____

Medication:_____For:_____ | P V H A E HO |

Dosage Info:_____Side Effects:_____

_____

Start Date:_____Stop Date:_____

Result?_____

Medication:_____For:_____ | P V H A E HO |

Dosage Info:_____Side Effects:_____

_____

Start Date:_____Stop Date:_____

Result?_____

P=Prescription, V=Vitamin, H=Herb, A=Amino Acid, E=Enzyme, HO=Homeopathic Remedy

Prescription Log

Medication:_____ For:_____ | P V H A E HO |

Dosage Info:_____ Side Effects:_____

_____

Start Date:_____ Stop Date:_____

Result?_____

Medication:_____ For:_____ | P V H A E HO |

Dosage Info:_____ Side Effects:_____

_____

Start Date:_____ Stop Date:_____

Result?_____

Medication:_____ For:_____ | P V H A E HO |

Dosage Info:_____ Side Effects:_____

_____

Start Date:_____ Stop Date:_____

Result?_____

Medication:_____ For:_____ | P V H A E HO |

Dosage Info:_____ Side Effects:_____

_____

Start Date:_____ Stop Date:_____

Result?_____

Medication:_____ For:_____ | P V H A E HO |

Dosage Info:_____ Side Effects:_____

_____

Start Date:_____ Stop Date:_____

Result?_____

| P=Prescription, V=Vitamin, H=Herb, A=Amino Acid, E=Enzyme, HO=Homeopathic Remedy |

Prescription Log

Medication:_____ For:_____ P V H A E HO

Dosage Info:_____ Side Effects:_____

_____

Start Date:_____ Stop Date:_____

Result?_____

Medication:_____ For:_____ P V H A E HO

Dosage Info:_____ Side Effects:_____

_____

Start Date:_____ Stop Date:_____

Result?_____

Medication:_____ For:_____ P V H A E HO

Dosage Info:_____ Side Effects:_____

_____

Start Date:_____ Stop Date:_____

Result?_____

Medication:_____ For:_____ P V H A E HO

Dosage Info:_____ Side Effects:_____

_____

Start Date:_____ Stop Date:_____

Result?_____

Medication:_____ For:_____ P V H A E HO

Dosage Info:_____ Side Effects:_____

_____

Start Date:_____ Stop Date:_____

Result?_____

P=Prescription, V=Vitamin, H=Herb, A=Amino Acid, E=Enzyme, HO=Homeopathic Remedy

OFFICE VISIT WORKSHEETS

Unless we are currently suffering from a chronic condition that forces us to be more diligent with our health, most of us put little thought into getting ready for a standard doctor appointment. Whatever the reason for your visit, preparing beforehand can help you get the most out of that visit. This preparation will also help your doctor to get necessary information from you to maintain your good health and may prevent serious illness in the future.

The most common appointment you will have with your doctor is your regular or annual check-up. Occasionally, a sudden minor illness brings you to your doctor sooner. Both these types of appointments are similarly prepared for and are not life-threatening situations. The information you gather at these appointments will help you and your doctor monitor trends in your health, so it will be important to you in the future to collect this information now, thus preventing possible health troubles later. Use the *Office Visit Worksheet* and *Vital Statistic Tracking Charts* in your handbook to monitor trends. Having this information organized for future use makes keeping control of your health quick and easy.

Your regular or annual check-up is the easiest appointment for which to prepare. The *Office Visit Worksheet* is designed especially for this type of appointment. The *Office Visit Worksheet* in your handbook can be kept up to date while you are waiting for your doctor. During your wait, simply jot down any questions you have been meaning to ask your doctor in the questions for this visit section of your *Office Visit Worksheet*. Review the *What Test At What Age Log* and note any tests that are suggested for your age to discuss with your doctor. Review the *Health History Summary Log*, note any tests that should be performed, and write down any questions you have about on-going prevention. In between visits, you may want to add questions for your upcoming appointments as they come to mind.

Following this section there are 30 *Office Visit Worksheets* and 5 of each *Vital Statistics Tracking Charts*.

Once you are in the examination room, the nurse or physician's assistant will take your temperature, weight and blood pressure. Collect this information from them and note it on your *Office Visit Worksheet* for transfer to your tracking chart. If you are tracking your cholesterol or blood sugar levels, note them on your *Office Visit Worksheet* and *Vital Statistic Tracking Charts* when you receive your test results. There are also four blank tracking spaces for you to use to track additional health condition indicators. If you DIY one of the blank tracking charts, take a minute to jot down the title of that tracking indicator on all your *Office Visit Worksheets* for future appointments or make a habit of glancing at your last *Office Visit Worksheet* during your waiting time. You do not want to forget to collect any important information.

The *Vital Statistic Tracking Charts* are where you will be notating the information from your office visits on an easy-to-understand visual graph. Your graph of vital statistics is an important tool for you and your doctor to see your health indicators at a glance. Keeping track of changes to your most important vital statistics helps you and your doctor when discussing what those changes mean to your health prevention plans. Coupled with the information you keep on your *Office Visit Worksheet* and your graph of vital statistics, both you and your doctor will become more proactive in maintaining your good health.

Your *Vital Statistics Tracking Charts* should be reviewed at each visit with your doctor. You and your doctor will use the vitals graph to track changes in your blood pressure, weight and cholesterol level. Additional blank graphs are there for you, as well. You can modify these graphs to track vital statistics that are more specific to your personal wellness program.

There are 5 copies of the *Weight/Body Fat Tracking Chart* starting on page 86. Many physicians are uncomfortable discussing weight gain with their patients. It is a sensitive subject for many people, and doctors may avoid discussing their patients' weight gain with them because they do not want to put their patients on the defensive. They, themselves, may be overweight and feel they would appear hypocritical discussing weight issues with you. Regardless of your feelings about weight, the reality is that each of us has a healthy weight range. If we stay within this range, we will have more success with our health. Maintaining a healthy weight promotes good health, making us less likely to develop weight-complicated illnesses, such as Type II diabetes, heart disease and high blood pressure. Your weight should be appropriate for your height, sex and fitness level. Look at the Body Mass Index (BMI) on page 85. Find your height and sex to determine your healthy BMI range. Place these numbers on your *Weight/Body Fat Tracking Chart.*

If you are very athletic or a body builder your BMI will not be correct. Because the BMI was designed for the *average* healthy person and does not take into account the heavier muscle weight of very fit individuals or bodybuilders. An alternative to the BMI would be to have your actual body fat measurements taken annually and use the Body Fat Chart / Body Mass Index to track that measurement. Determine with the help of your doctor a healthy body fat level for you.

There are 5 copies of the *Blood Pressure Tracking Chart* starting on page 91. Most office visits include a blood pressure reading. High blood pressure can be a warning sign of a variety of conditions. Your blood pressure reading is made up of two components: Systolic pressure and diastolic pressure. The systolic readings are considered normal when they fall below 130. Diastolic readings are considered normal when they fall below 80. The blood pressure chart tracks both of these normal ranges in gray shading. Fill in the readings at each visit and discuss any unusual movement with your doctor.

There are 5 copies of the *Cholesterol Tracking Chart* starting on page 96. Cholesterol readings are not often taken during your regular office visits. Some doctors consider high cholesterol levels as an indicator of future problems of the heart and arteries. Recent research regarding Cholesterol is changing our view of Cholesterol and some research has found that individuals with higher levels show no signs of heart and artery disease. For Cholesterol testing you may want to work closely with your doctor based on your personal history to develop a useful testing schedule. Use the *Cholesterol Tracking Chart* to monitor your cholesterol readings.

There are 5 *Blank Tracking Charts* starting on page 101. If you have an illness that requires you to be tested regularly, and those readings are indicators of your well-being then use the blank tracking graphs. To create a personalized graph, first discuss the range of normal for the indicator you wish to track with your doctor, then use that range to create your graph and monitor your progress. If you highlight the range of normal on your graph with a highlighter marker, it is much easier to see when you fall outside of the normal range.

As an example, you could use a blank tracking graph to monitor headaches or other types of pain. Use the graph as a pain scale by assigning a scale from 1-10. When pain occurs, write in the date and mark the degree of pain as it applies to your scale. With this kind of pain tracking, you and your doctor can determine if the attacks are getting closer together, becoming more severe, or are falling into a pattern. For more serious on-going symptoms, use the *Detection Worksheet* on page 107. The *Detection Worksheet* is designed to track your symptoms in more detail than the graphs do and can be used alone or along with the graphs as an important diagnostic tool for you and your doctor.

It is easier to make minor lifestyle and diet changes before your health gets outside of the range of normal. By maintaining a vital statistics graph, and taking more control of your health you may be better able to tackle a problem before it becomes serious enough to require medication, and more drastic lifestyle and dietary changes.

A sudden minor illness appointment is also very easy to prepare for by using the *Office Visit Worksheets*. Again, while you are sitting in the waiting room, make note of any questions you may have for your doctor in the questions section.

List all your symptoms in the Symptoms section. Jot down any remedies or over-the-counter medicines you have already tried and the results you have had with them. Use the figure to identify problem areas, by placing an "X" to mark the spot and circle the type of pain. Or write the letter on the figure where you are experiencing that type of pain. The better you can describe what is going on inside you, the better your diagnosis will be.

Write in any tests taken on this visit and the Doctors recommendations. Then note the results of your tests and the advices given once that information is known.

You can leave the test/result information here in the *Office Visit Worksheet* or transfer the information over to your *What Tests at What Age Log* so it's available at a glance.

If you are given a prescription, add that to your prescription log so you can track when to start and stop that remedy, how it performs for your condition and any side-effects you might experience.

Office Visit Worksheet

Date_____Reason for Visit:_____Doctor:_____

Weight:_____Temperature:_____Blood Pressure Reading:_____over_____

If Blood Sugar & Cholesterol Testing was done

Blood Sugar:_____Fasted or Not? _____

Cholesterol Total:_____HDL:_____LDL:_____Triglycerides:_____Fasted or Not?_____

Additional readings from other tests specific to you

Test:_____Result:_____Test:_____Result:_____

Test:_____Result:_____Test:_____Result:_____

Symptoms:_____

_____

Treatments Tried at home:_____Results:_____

Treatment Recommended at this visit:_____Results:_____

Questions for this visit: *use previous visit sheets as a reminder of any unfinished discussions.*_____

_____

_____

_____

Tests Suggested by Age:_____

_____

_____

Tests Suggested by Health History: _____

_____

_____

Tests Recommended or Performed for Today's Diagnosis:_____

_____

_____

(Note all tests and test results on your test results log or tracking chart)

Pain Type & Location:	Doctor recommendations for this visit:
S-Sharp T-Throbbing C-Constant	
R-Radiating M-With Movement	
AM PM All Day Day & Night	
	Results:

Office Visit Worksheet

Date_____Reason for Visit:_____Doctor:_____

Weight:_____Temperature:_____Blood Pressure Reading:_____over_____

If Blood Sugar & Cholesterol Testing was done

Blood Sugar:_____Fasted or Not? _____

Cholesterol Total:_____HDL:_____LDL:_____Triglycerides:_____Fasted or Not?_____

Additional readings from other tests specific to you

Test:_____Result:_____Test:_____Result:_____

Test:_____Result:_____Test:_____Result:_____

Symptoms:_____

_____

Treatments Tried at home:_____Results:_____

Treatment Recommended at this visit:_____Results:_____

Questions for this visit: *use previous visit sheets as a reminder of any unfinished discussions.*_____

_____

_____

_____

Tests Suggested by Age:_____

_____

Tests Suggested by Health History: _____

_____

Tests Recommended or Performed for Today's Diagnosis:_____

_____

(Note all tests and test results on your test results log or tracking chart)

Pain Type & Location:	Doctor recommendations for this visit:
S-Sharp T-Throbbing C-Constant	
R-Radiating M-With Movement	
AM PM All Day Day & Night	
	Results:

Office Visit Worksheet

Date_____Reason for Visit:_____Doctor:_____

Weight:_____Temperature:_____Blood Pressure Reading:_____over_____

If Blood Sugar & Cholesterol Testing was done

Blood Sugar:_____Fasted or Not? _____

Cholesterol Total:_____HDL:_____LDL:_____Triglycerides:_____Fasted or Not?_____

Additional readings from other tests specific to you

Test:_____Result:_____Test:_____Result:_____

Test:_____Result:_____Test:_____Result:_____

Symptoms:_____

_____

Treatments Tried at home:_____Results:_____

Treatment Recommended at this visit:_____Results:_____

Questions for this visit: *use previous visit sheets as a reminder of any unfinished discussions.*_____

_____

_____

_____

Tests Suggested by Age:_____

_____

Tests Suggested by Health History: _____

_____

Tests Recommended or Performed for Today's Diagnosis:_____

_____

(Note all tests and test results on your test results log or tracking chart)

Pain Type & Location:	Doctor recommendations for this visit:
S-Sharp T-Throbbing C-Constant	
R-Radiating M-With Movement	
AM PM All Day Day & Night	
	Results:

Office Visit Worksheet

Date_____Reason for Visit:_____Doctor:_____
Weight:_____Temperature:_____Blood Pressure Reading:_____over_____
If Blood Sugar & Cholesterol Testing was done
Blood Sugar:_____Fasted or Not? _____
Cholesterol Total:_____HDL:_____LDL:_____Triglycerides:_____Fasted or Not?_____
Additional readings from other tests specific to you
Test:_____Result:_____Test:_____Result:_____
Test:_____Result:_____Test:_____Result:_____

Symptoms:_____
_____
Treatments Tried at home:_____Results:_____
Treatment Recommended at this visit:_____Results:_____

Questions for this visit: *use previous visit sheets as a reminder of any unfinished discussions.*_____
_____
_____
_____

Tests Suggested by Age:_____
_____
_____

Tests Suggested by Health History: _____
_____
_____

Tests Recommended or Performed for Today's Diagnosis:_____
_____
_____

(Note all tests and test results on your test results log or tracking chart)

Pain Type & Location:	Doctor recommendations for this visit:
S-Sharp T-Throbbing C-Constant	
R-Radiating M-With Movement	
AM PM All Day Day & Night	
	Results:

Office Visit Worksheet

Date_____Reason for Visit:_____Doctor:_____

Weight:_____Temperature:_____Blood Pressure Reading:_____over_____

If Blood Sugar & Cholesterol Testing was done

Blood Sugar:_____Fasted or Not? _____

Cholesterol Total:_____HDL:_____LDL:_____Triglycerides:_____Fasted or Not?_____

Additional readings from other tests specific to you

Test:_____Result:_____Test:_____Result:_____

Test:_____Result:_____Test:_____Result:_____

Symptoms:_____

_____

Treatments Tried at home:_____Results:_____

Treatment Recommended at this visit:_____Results:_____

Questions for this visit: *use previous visit sheets as a reminder of any unfinished discussions.*_____

_____

_____

_____

Tests Suggested by Age:_____

_____

Tests Suggested by Health History: _____

_____

Tests Recommended or Performed for Today's Diagnosis:_____

_____

(Note all tests and test results on your test results log or tracking chart)

Pain Type & Location:	Doctor recommendations for this visit:
S-Sharp T-Throbbing C-Constant	
R-Radiating M-With Movement	
AM PM All Day Day & Night	
	Results:

Office Visit Worksheet

Date_____Reason for Visit:_____Doctor:_____
Weight:_____Temperature:_____Blood Pressure Reading:_____over_____

If Blood Sugar & Cholesterol Testing was done
Blood Sugar:_____Fasted or Not? _____
Cholesterol Total:_____HDL:_____LDL:_____Triglycerides:_____Fasted or Not?_____

Additional readings from other tests specific to you
Test:_____Result:_____Test:_____Result:_____
Test:_____Result:_____Test:_____Result:_____

Symptoms:_____
_____
Treatments Tried at home:_____Results:_____
Treatment Recommended at this visit:_____Results:_____

Questions for this visit: *use previous visit sheets as a reminder of any unfinished discussions.*
_____
_____
_____

Tests Suggested by Age:_____
_____

Tests Suggested by Health History: _____
_____

Tests Recommended or Performed for Today's Diagnosis:_____
_____
_____

(Note all tests and test results on your test results log or tracking chart)

Pain Type & Location:	Doctor recommendations for this visit:
S-Sharp T-Throbbing C-Constant	
R-Radiating M-With Movement	
AM PM All Day Day & Night	
	Results:

Office Visit Worksheet

Date_____Reason for Visit:_____Doctor:_____

Weight:_____Temperature:_____Blood Pressure Reading:_____over_____

If Blood Sugar & Cholesterol Testing was done

Blood Sugar:_____Fasted or Not? _____

Cholesterol Total:_____HDL:_____LDL:_____Triglycerides:_____Fasted or Not?_____

Additional readings from other tests specific to you

Test:_____Result:_____Test:_____Result:_____

Test:_____Result:_____Test:_____Result:_____

Symptoms:_____

_____

Treatments Tried at home:_____Results:_____

Treatment Recommended at this visit:_____Results:_____

Questions for this visit: *use previous visit sheets as a reminder of any unfinished discussions.*_____

_____

_____

_____

Tests Suggested by Age:_____

_____

Tests Suggested by Health History: _____

_____

Tests Recommended or Performed for Today's Diagnosis:_____

_____

(Note all tests and test results on your test results log or tracking chart)

Pain Type & Location:	Doctor recommendations for this visit:
S-Sharp T-Throbbing C-Constant	
R-Radiating M-With Movement	
AM PM All Day Day & Night	
	Results:

Office Visit Worksheet

Date_____Reason for Visit:_____Doctor:_____

Weight:_____Temperature:_____Blood Pressure Reading:_____over_____

If Blood Sugar & Cholesterol Testing was done

Blood Sugar:_____Fasted or Not? _____

Cholesterol Total:_____HDL:_____LDL:_____Triglycerides:_____Fasted or Not?_____

Additional readings from other tests specific to you

Test:_____Result:_____Test:_____Result:_____

Test:_____Result:_____Test:_____Result:_____

Symptoms:_____

_____

Treatments Tried at home:_____Results:_____

Treatment Recommended at this visit:_____Results:_____

Questions for this visit: *use previous visit sheets as a reminder of any unfinished discussions.*_____

_____

_____

_____

Tests Suggested by Age:_____

_____

_____

Tests Suggested by Health History: _____

_____

Tests Recommended or Performed for Today's Diagnosis:_____

_____

_____

(Note all tests and test results on your test results log or tracking chart)

Pain Type & Location:	Doctor recommendations for this visit:
S-Sharp T-Throbbing C-Constant	
R-Radiating M-With Movement	
AM PM All Day Day & Night	
	Results:

Office Visit Worksheet

Date_____Reason for Visit:_____Doctor:_____

Weight:_____Temperature:_____Blood Pressure Reading:_____ over_____

If Blood Sugar & Cholesterol Testing was done

Blood Sugar:_____Fasted or Not? _____

Cholesterol Total:_____HDL:_____LDL:_____Triglycerides:_____Fasted or Not?_____

Additional readings from other tests specific to you

Test:_____Result:_____Test:_____Result:_____

Test:_____Result:_____Test:_____Result:_____

Symptoms:_____

_____

Treatments Tried at home:_____Results:_____

Treatment Recommended at this visit:_____Results:_____

Questions for this visit: *use previous visit sheets as a reminder of any unfinished discussions.*_____

_____

_____

_____

Tests Suggested by Age:_____

_____

_____

Tests Suggested by Health History: _____

_____

_____

Tests Recommended or Performed for Today's Diagnosis:_____

_____

_____

(Note all tests and test results on your test results log or tracking chart)

Pain Type & Location:	Doctor recommendations for this visit:
S-Sharp T-Throbbing C-Constant	
R-Radiating M-With Movement	
AM PM All Day Day & Night	
	Results:

Office Visit Worksheet

Date_____Reason for Visit:_____Doctor:_____

Weight:_____Temperature:_____Blood Pressure Reading:_____over_____

If Blood Sugar & Cholesterol Testing was done

Blood Sugar:_____Fasted or Not? _____

Cholesterol Total:_____HDL:_____LDL:_____Triglycerides:_____Fasted or Not?_____

Additional readings from other tests specific to you

Test:_____Result:_____Test:_____Result:_____

Test:_____Result:_____Test:_____Result:_____

Symptoms:_____

_____

Treatments Tried at home:_____Results:_____

Treatment Recommended at this visit:_____Results:_____

Questions for this visit: *use previous visit sheets as a reminder of any unfinished discussions.*_____

_____

_____

_____

Tests Suggested by Age:_____

_____

Tests Suggested by Health History: _____

_____

Tests Recommended or Performed for Today's Diagnosis:_____

_____

_____

(Note all tests and test results on your test results log or tracking chart)

Pain Type & Location:	Doctor recommendations for this visit:
S-Sharp T-Throbbing C-Constant	
R-Radiating M-With Movement	
AM PM All Day Day & Night	
	Results:

Office Visit Worksheet

Date_____Reason for Visit:_____Doctor:_____

Weight:_____Temperature:_____Blood Pressure Reading:_____over_____

If Blood Sugar & Cholesterol Testing was done

Blood Sugar:_____Fasted or Not? _____

Cholesterol Total:_____HDL:_____LDL:_____Triglycerides:_____Fasted or Not?_____

Additional readings from other tests specific to you

Test:_____Result:_____Test:_____Result:_____

Test:_____Result:_____Test:_____Result:_____

Symptoms:_____

_____

Treatments Tried at home:_____Results:_____

Treatment Recommended at this visit:_____Results:_____

Questions for this visit: *use previous visit sheets as a reminder of any unfinished discussions.*_____

_____

_____

_____

Tests Suggested by Age:_____

_____

_____

Tests Suggested by Health History: _____

_____

_____

Tests Recommended or Performed for Today's Diagnosis:_____

_____

_____

(Note all tests and test results on your test results log or tracking chart)

Pain Type & Location:	Doctor recommendations for this visit:
S-Sharp T-Throbbing C-Constant	
R-Radiating M-With Movement	
AM PM All Day Day & Night	
	Results:

Office Visit Worksheet

Date_____Reason for Visit:_____Doctor:_____

Weight:_____Temperature:_____Blood Pressure Reading:_____over_____

If Blood Sugar & Cholesterol Testing was done

Blood Sugar:_____Fasted or Not? _____

Cholesterol Total:_____HDL:_____LDL:_____Triglycerides:_____Fasted or Not?_____

Additional readings from other tests specific to you

Test:_____Result:_____Test:_____Result:_____

Test:_____Result:_____Test:_____Result:_____

Symptoms:_____

_____

Treatments Tried at home:_____Results:_____

Treatment Recommended at this visit:_____Results:_____

Questions for this visit: *use previous visit sheets as a reminder of any unfinished discussions.*_____

_____

_____

_____

Tests Suggested by Age:_____

_____

Tests Suggested by Health History: _____

_____

Tests Recommended or Performed for Today's Diagnosis:_____

_____

(Note all tests and test results on your test results log or tracking chart)

Pain Type & Location:	Doctor recommendations for this visit:
S-Sharp T-Throbbing C-Constant	
R-Radiating M-With Movement	
AM PM All Day Day & Night	
	Results:

Office Visit Worksheet

Date_____Reason for Visit:_____Doctor:_____

Weight:_____Temperature:_____Blood Pressure Reading:_____over_____

If Blood Sugar & Cholesterol Testing was done

Blood Sugar:_____Fasted or Not? _____

Cholesterol Total:_____HDL:_____LDL:_____Triglycerides:_____Fasted or Not?_____

Additional readings from other tests specific to you

Test:_____Result:_____Test:_____Result:_____

Test:_____Result:_____Test:_____Result:_____

Symptoms:_____

_____

Treatments Tried at home:_____Results:_____

Treatment Recommended at this visit:_____Results:_____

Questions for this visit: *use previous visit sheets as a reminder of any unfinished discussions.*_____

_____

_____

_____

Tests Suggested by Age:_____

_____

Tests Suggested by Health History: _____

_____

Tests Recommended or Performed for Today's Diagnosis:_____

_____

(Note all tests and test results on your test results log or tracking chart)

Pain Type & Location:	Doctor recommendations for this visit:
S-Sharp T-Throbbing C-Constant	
R-Radiating M-With Movement	
AM PM All Day Day & Night	
	Results:

66

Office Visit Worksheet

Date_____Reason for Visit:_____Doctor:_____

Weight:_____Temperature:_____Blood Pressure Reading:_____over_____

If Blood Sugar & Cholesterol Testing was done

Blood Sugar:_____Fasted or Not? _____

Cholesterol Total:_____HDL:_____LDL:_____Triglycerides:_____Fasted or Not?_____

Additional readings from other tests specific to you

Test:_____Result:_____Test:_____Result:_____

Test:_____Result:_____Test:_____Result:_____

Symptoms:_____

_____

Treatments Tried at home:_____Results:_____

Treatment Recommended at this visit:_____Results:_____

Questions for this visit: *use previous visit sheets as a reminder of any unfinished discussions.*_____

_____

_____

_____

Tests Suggested by Age:_____

_____

_____

Tests Suggested by Health History: _____

_____

_____

Tests Recommended or Performed for Today's Diagnosis:_____

_____

_____

(Note all tests and test results on your test results log or tracking chart)

Pain Type & Location:	Doctor recommendations for this visit:
S-Sharp T-Throbbing C-Constant	
R-Radiating M-With Movement	
AM PM All Day Day & Night	
	Results:

Office Visit Worksheet

Date_____Reason for Visit:_____Doctor:_____

Weight:_____Temperature:_____Blood Pressure Reading:_____over_____

If Blood Sugar & Cholesterol Testing was done

Blood Sugar:_____Fasted or Not? _____

Cholesterol Total:_____HDL:_____LDL:_____Triglycerides:_____Fasted or Not?_____

Additional readings from other tests specific to you

Test:_____Result:_____Test:_____Result:_____

Test:_____Result:_____Test:_____Result:_____

Symptoms:_____

_____

Treatments Tried at home:_____Results:_____

Treatment Recommended at this visit:_____Results:_____

Questions for this visit: *use previous visit sheets as a reminder of any unfinished discussions.*_____

_____

_____

_____

Tests Suggested by Age:_____

_____

Tests Suggested by Health History: _____

_____

Tests Recommended or Performed for Today's Diagnosis:_____

_____

(Note all tests and test results on your test results log or tracking chart)

Pain Type & Location:	Doctor recommendations for this visit:
S-Sharp T-Throbbing C-Constant	
R-Radiating M-With Movement	
AM PM All Day Day & Night	
	Results:

Office Visit Worksheet

Date_____Reason for Visit:_____Doctor:_____
Weight:_____Temperature:_____Blood Pressure Reading:_____over _____
If Blood Sugar & Cholesterol Testing was done
Blood Sugar:_____Fasted or Not? _____
Cholesterol Total:_____HDL:_____LDL:_____Triglycerides:_____Fasted or Not?_____
Additional readings from other tests specific to you
Test:_____Result:_____Test:_____Result:_____
Test:_____Result:_____Test:_____Result:_____

Symptoms:_____
_____
Treatments Tried at home:_____Results:_____
Treatment Recommended at this visit:_____Results:_____

Questions for this visit: *use previous visit sheets as a reminder of any unfinished discussions.*_____
_____
_____
_____

Tests Suggested by Age:_____
_____
_____

Tests Suggested by Health History: _____
_____
_____

Tests Recommended or Performed for Today's Diagnosis:_____
_____
_____

(Note all tests and test results on your test results log or tracking chart)

Pain Type & Location:	Doctor recommendations for this visit:
S-Sharp T-Throbbing C-Constant	
R-Radiating M-With Movement	
AM PM All Day Day & Night	
	Results:

Office Visit Worksheet

Date_____Reason for Visit:_____Doctor:_____

Weight:_____Temperature:_____Blood Pressure Reading:_____ over _____

If Blood Sugar & Cholesterol Testing was done

Blood Sugar:_____Fasted or Not? _____

Cholesterol Total:_____HDL:_____LDL:_____Triglycerides:_____Fasted or Not?_____

Additional readings from other tests specific to you

Test:_____Result:_____Test:_____Result:_____

Test:_____Result:_____Test:_____Result:_____

Symptoms:_____

_____

Treatments Tried at home:_____Results:_____

Treatment Recommended at this visit:_____Results:_____

Questions for this visit: *use previous visit sheets as a reminder of any unfinished discussions.*_____

_____

_____

_____

_____

Tests Suggested by Age:_____

_____

_____

Tests Suggested by Health History: _____

_____

_____

Tests Recommended or Performed for Today's Diagnosis:_____

_____

_____

(Note all tests and test results on your test results log or tracking chart)

Pain Type & Location:	Doctor recommendations for this visit:
S-Sharp T-Throbbing C-Constant	
R-Radiating M-With Movement	
AM PM All Day Day & Night	
	Results:

Office Visit Worksheet

Date_____Reason for Visit:_____Doctor:_____

Weight:_____Temperature:_____Blood Pressure Reading:_____over_____

If Blood Sugar & Cholesterol Testing was done

Blood Sugar:_____Fasted or Not? _____

Cholesterol Total:_____HDL:_____LDL:_____Triglycerides:_____Fasted or Not?_____

Additional readings from other tests specific to you

Test:_____Result:_____Test:_____Result:_____

Test:_____Result:_____Test:_____Result:_____

Symptoms:_____

_____

Treatments Tried at home:_____Results:_____

Treatment Recommended at this visit:_____Results:_____

Questions for this visit: *use previous visit sheets as a reminder of any unfinished discussions.*_____

_____

_____

_____

Tests Suggested by Age:_____

_____

_____

Tests Suggested by Health History: _____

_____

_____

Tests Recommended or Performed for Today's Diagnosis:_____

_____

_____

(Note all tests and test results on your test results log or tracking chart)

Pain Type & Location:	Doctor recommendations for this visit:
S-Sharp T-Throbbing C-Constant	
R-Radiating M-With Movement	
AM PM All Day Day & Night	
	Results:

Office Visit Worksheet

Date_____Reason for Visit:_____Doctor:_____
Weight:_____Temperature:_____Blood Pressure Reading:_____over_____
If Blood Sugar & Cholesterol Testing was done
Blood Sugar:_____Fasted or Not? _____
Cholesterol Total:_____HDL:_____LDL:_____Triglycerides:_____Fasted or Not?_____
Additional readings from other tests specific to you
Test:_____Result:_____Test:_____Result:_____
Test:_____Result:_____Test:_____Result:_____

Symptoms:_____
_____
Treatments Tried at home:_____Results:_____
Treatment Recommended at this visit:_____Results:_____

Questions for this visit: *use previous visit sheets as a reminder of any unfinished discussions.*_____
_____
_____
_____

Tests Suggested by Age:_____
_____

Tests Suggested by Health History: _____
_____

Tests Recommended or Performed for Today's Diagnosis:_____
_____

(Note all tests and test results on your test results log or tracking chart)

Pain Type & Location:	Doctor recommendations for this visit:
S-Sharp T-Throbbing C-Constant	
R-Radiating M-With Movement	
AM PM All Day Day & Night	
	Results:

Office Visit Worksheet

Date_____Reason for Visit:_____Doctor:_____

Weight:_____Temperature:_____Blood Pressure Reading:_____over_____

If Blood Sugar & Cholesterol Testing was done

Blood Sugar:_____Fasted or Not? _____

Cholesterol Total:_____HDL:_____LDL:_____Triglycerides:_____Fasted or Not?_____

Additional readings from other tests specific to you

Test:_____Result:_____Test:_____Result:_____

Test:_____Result:_____Test:_____Result:_____

Symptoms:_____

_____

Treatments Tried at home:_____Results:_____

Treatment Recommended at this visit:_____Results:_____

Questions for this visit: *use previous visit sheets as a reminder of any unfinished discussions.*_____

_____

_____

_____

Tests Suggested by Age:_____

_____

Tests Suggested by Health History: _____

_____

Tests Recommended or Performed for Today's Diagnosis:_____

_____

(Note all tests and test results on your test results log or tracking chart)

Pain Type & Location:	Doctor recommendations for this visit:
S-Sharp T-Throbbing C-Constant	
R-Radiating M-With Movement	
AM PM All Day Day & Night	
	Results:

Office Visit Worksheet

Date_____Reason for Visit:_____Doctor:_____
Weight:_____Temperature:_____Blood Pressure Reading:_____over_____
If Blood Sugar & Cholesterol Testing was done
Blood Sugar:_____Fasted or Not? _____
Cholesterol Total:_____HDL:_____LDL:_____Triglycerides:_____Fasted or Not?_____
Additional readings from other tests specific to you
Test:_____Result:_____Test:_____Result:_____
Test:_____Result:_____Test:_____Result:_____

Symptoms:_____
_____
Treatments Tried at home:_____Results:_____
Treatment Recommended at this visit:_____Results:_____

Questions for this visit: *use previous visit sheets as a reminder of any unfinished discussions.*_____
_____
_____
_____

Tests Suggested by Age:_____
_____
_____
Tests Suggested by Health History: _____
_____
_____
Tests Recommended or Performed for Today's Diagnosis:_____
_____
_____

(Note all tests and test results on your test results log or tracking chart)

Pain Type & Location:	Doctor recommendations for this visit:
S-Sharp T-Throbbing C-Constant	
R-Radiating M-With Movement	
AM PM All Day Day & Night	
	Results:

Office Visit Worksheet

Date_____Reason for Visit:_____Doctor:_____

Weight:_____Temperature:_____Blood Pressure Reading:_____over_____

If Blood Sugar & Cholesterol Testing was done

Blood Sugar:_____Fasted or Not? _____

Cholesterol Total:_____HDL:_____LDL:_____Triglycerides:_____Fasted or Not?_____

Additional readings from other tests specific to you

Test:_____Result:_____Test:_____Result:_____

Test:_____Result:_____Test:_____Result:_____

Symptoms:_____

_____

Treatments Tried at home:_____Results:_____

Treatment Recommended at this visit:_____Results:_____

Questions for this visit: *use previous visit sheets as a reminder of any unfinished discussions.*_____

_____

_____

_____

Tests Suggested by Age:_____

_____

Tests Suggested by Health History: _____

_____

Tests Recommended or Performed for Today's Diagnosis:_____

_____

(Note all tests and test results on your test results log or tracking chart)

Pain Type & Location:	Doctor recommendations for this visit:
S-Sharp T-Throbbing C-Constant	
R-Radiating M-With Movement	
AM PM All Day Day & Night	
	Results:

Office Visit Worksheet

Date_____Reason for Visit:_____Doctor:_____
Weight:_____Temperature:_____Blood Pressure Reading:_____over_____
If Blood Sugar & Cholesterol Testing was done
Blood Sugar:_____Fasted or Not? _____
Cholesterol Total:_____HDL:_____LDL:_____Triglycerides:_____Fasted or Not?_____
Additional readings from other tests specific to you
Test:_____Result:_____Test:_____Result:_____
Test:_____Result:_____Test:_____Result:_____

Symptoms:_____
_____
Treatments Tried at home:_____Results:_____
Treatment Recommended at this visit:_____Results:_____

Questions for this visit: *use previous visit sheets as a reminder of any unfinished discussions.*_____
_____
_____
_____

Tests Suggested by Age:_____
_____
_____

Tests Suggested by Health History: _____
_____
_____

Tests Recommended or Performed for Today's Diagnosis:_____
_____
_____

(Note all tests and test results on your test results log or tracking chart)

Pain Type & Location:	Doctor recommendations for this visit:
S-Sharp T-Throbbing C-Constant	
R-Radiating M-With Movement	
AM PM All Day Day & Night	
	Results:

Office Visit Worksheet

Date_____Reason for Visit:_____Doctor:_____
Weight:_____Temperature:_____Blood Pressure Reading:_____over_____
If Blood Sugar & Cholesterol Testing was done
Blood Sugar:_____Fasted or Not? _____
Cholesterol Total:_____HDL:_____LDL:_____Triglycerides:_____Fasted or Not?_____
Additional readings from other tests specific to you
Test:_____Result:_____Test:_____Result:_____
Test:_____Result:_____Test:_____Result:_____

Symptoms:_____
_____
Treatments Tried at home:_____Results:_____
Treatment Recommended at this visit:_____Results:_____

Questions for this visit: *use previous visit sheets as a reminder of any unfinished discussions.*_____
_____
_____
_____

Tests Suggested by Age:_____
_____

Tests Suggested by Health History: _____
_____

Tests Recommended or Performed for Today's Diagnosis:_____
_____

(Note all tests and test results on your test results log or tracking chart)

Pain Type & Location:	Doctor recommendations for this visit:
S-Sharp T-Throbbing C-Constant	
R-Radiating M-With Movement	
AM PM All Day Day & Night	
	Results:

Office Visit Worksheet

Date_____Reason for Visit:_____Doctor:_____

Weight:_____Temperature:_____Blood Pressure Reading:_____over_____

If Blood Sugar & Cholesterol Testing was done

Blood Sugar:_____Fasted or Not? _____

Cholesterol Total:_____HDL:_____LDL:_____Triglycerides:_____Fasted or Not?_____

Additional readings from other tests specific to you

Test:_____Result:_____Test:_____Result:_____

Test:_____Result:_____Test:_____Result:_____

Symptoms:_____

_____

Treatments Tried at home:_____Results:_____

Treatment Recommended at this visit:_____Results:_____

Questions for this visit: *use previous visit sheets as a reminder of any unfinished discussions.*_____

_____

_____

_____

Tests Suggested by Age:_____

_____

_____

Tests Suggested by Health History: _____

_____

Tests Recommended or Performed for Today's Diagnosis:_____

_____

_____

(Note all tests and test results on your test results log or tracking chart)

Pain Type & Location:	Doctor recommendations for this visit:
S-Sharp T-Throbbing C-Constant	
R-Radiating M-With Movement	
AM PM All Day Day & Night	
	Results:

Office Visit Worksheet

Date_____Reason for Visit:_____Doctor:_____

Weight:_____Temperature:_____Blood Pressure Reading:_____over_____

If Blood Sugar & Cholesterol Testing was done

Blood Sugar:_____Fasted or Not? _____

Cholesterol Total:_____HDL:_____LDL:_____Triglycerides:_____Fasted or Not?_____

Additional readings from other tests specific to you

Test:_____Result:_____Test:_____Result:_____

Test:_____Result:_____Test:_____Result:_____

Symptoms:_____

_____

Treatments Tried at home:_____Results:_____

Treatment Recommended at this visit:_____Results:_____

Questions for this visit: *use previous visit sheets as a reminder of any unfinished discussions.*

_____

_____

_____

Tests Suggested by Age:_____

_____

Tests Suggested by Health History: _____

_____

Tests Recommended or Performed for Today's Diagnosis:_____

_____

_____

(Note all tests and test results on your test results log or tracking chart)

Pain Type & Location:	Doctor recommendations for this visit:
S-Sharp T-Throbbing C-Constant	
R-Radiating M-With Movement	
AM PM All Day Day & Night	
	Results:

Office Visit Worksheet

Date_____Reason for Visit:_____Doctor:_____

Weight:_____Temperature:_____Blood Pressure Reading:_____ over _____

If Blood Sugar & Cholesterol Testing was done

Blood Sugar:_____Fasted or Not? _____

Cholesterol Total:_____HDL:_____LDL:_____Triglycerides:_____Fasted or Not?_____

Additional readings from other tests specific to you

Test:_____Result:_____Test:_____Result:_____

Test:_____Result:_____Test:_____Result:_____

Symptoms:_____

_____

Treatments Tried at home:_____Results:_____

Treatment Recommended at this visit:_____Results:_____

Questions for this visit: *use previous visit sheets as a reminder of any unfinished discussions.*_____

_____

_____

_____

Tests Suggested by Age:_____

_____

_____

Tests Suggested by Health History: _____

_____

_____

Tests Recommended or Performed for Today's Diagnosis:_____

_____

_____

(Note all tests and test results on your test results log or tracking chart)

Pain Type & Location:	Doctor recommendations for this visit:
S-Sharp T-Throbbing C-Constant	
R-Radiating M-With Movement	
AM PM All Day Day & Night	
	Results:

Office Visit Worksheet

Date_____Reason for Visit:_____Doctor:_____

Weight:_____Temperature:_____Blood Pressure Reading:_____over_____

If Blood Sugar & Cholesterol Testing was done

Blood Sugar:_____Fasted or Not? _____

Cholesterol Total:_____HDL:_____LDL:_____Triglycerides:_____Fasted or Not?_____

Additional readings from other tests specific to you

Test:_____Result:_____Test:_____Result:_____

Test:_____Result:_____Test:_____Result:_____

Symptoms:_____

_____

Treatments Tried at home:_____Results:_____

Treatment Recommended at this visit:_____Results:_____

Questions for this visit: *use previous visit sheets as a reminder of any unfinished discussions.*_____

_____

_____

_____

Tests Suggested by Age:_____

_____

Tests Suggested by Health History: _____

_____

Tests Recommended or Performed for Today's Diagnosis:_____

_____

_____

(Note all tests and test results on your test results log or tracking chart)

Pain Type & Location:	Doctor recommendations for this visit:
S-Sharp T-Throbbing C-Constant	
R-Radiating M-With Movement	
AM PM All Day Day & Night	
	Results:

Office Visit Worksheet

Date_____Reason for Visit:_____Doctor:_____

Weight:_____Temperature:_____Blood Pressure Reading:_____over_____

If Blood Sugar & Cholesterol Testing was done

Blood Sugar:_____Fasted or Not? _____

Cholesterol Total:_____HDL:_____LDL:_____Triglycerides:_____Fasted or Not?_____

Additional readings from other tests specific to you

Test:_____Result:_____Test:_____Result:_____

Test:_____Result:_____Test:_____Result:_____

Symptoms:_____

_____

Treatments Tried at home:_____Results:_____

Treatment Recommended at this visit:_____Results:_____

Questions for this visit: *use previous visit sheets as a reminder of any unfinished discussions.*_____

_____

_____

_____

Tests Suggested by Age:_____

_____

Tests Suggested by Health History: _____

_____

Tests Recommended or Performed for Today's Diagnosis:_____

_____

_____

(Note all tests and test results on your test results log or tracking chart)

Pain Type & Location:	Doctor recommendations for this visit:
S-Sharp T-Throbbing C-Constant	
R-Radiating M-With Movement	
AM PM All Day Day & Night	
	Results:

Office Visit Worksheet

Date_____Reason for Visit:_____Doctor:_____
Weight:_____Temperature:_____Blood Pressure Reading:_____over_____
If Blood Sugar & Cholesterol Testing was done
Blood Sugar:_____Fasted or Not? _____
Cholesterol Total:_____HDL:_____LDL:_____Triglycerides:_____Fasted or Not?_____
Additional readings from other tests specific to you
Test:_____Result:_____Test:_____Result:_____
Test:_____Result:_____Test:_____Result:_____

Symptoms:_____
_____
Treatments Tried at home:_____Results:_____
Treatment Recommended at this visit:_____Results:_____

Questions for this visit: *use previous visit sheets as a reminder of any unfinished discussions.*
_____
_____
_____
_____

Tests Suggested by Age:_____
_____
_____
Tests Suggested by Health History: _____
_____
_____
Tests Recommended or Performed for Today's Diagnosis:_____
_____
_____

(Note all tests and test results on your test results log or tracking chart)

Pain Type & Location:	Doctor recommendations for this visit:
S-Sharp T-Throbbing C-Constant	
R-Radiating M-With Movement	
AM PM All Day Day & Night	
	Results:

NOTES:

Body Mass Index Chart and Risk Assessment

BMI	19	20	21	22	23	24	25	26	27	28	29	30	35	40
Height In Inches			Normal Range						Increased Risk			Danger Range		
58	91	96	100	105	110	115	119	124	129	134	138	143	167	191
59	94	99	104	109	114	119	124	128	133	138	143	148	173	198
60	97	102	107	112	118	123	128	133	138	143	148	153	179	204
61	100	106	111	116	122	127	132	137	143	148	153	158	185	211
62	104	109	115	120	126	131	136	142	147	153	158	164	191	218
63	107	113	118	124	130	135	141	146	152	158	163	159	197	225
64	110	116	122	128	134	140	145	151	157	163	169	174	204	232
65	114	120	126	132	128	144	150	156	162	168	174	180	210	240
66	118	124	130	136	142	148	155	161	167	173	179	186	216	247
67	121	127	134	140	146	153	159	166	172	178	185	191	223	255
68	125	131	138	144	151	158	164	171	177	184	190	197	230	262
69	128	165	142	149	155	162	169	176	182	189	196	203	236	270
70	132	139	146	153	160	167	147	181	188	195	202	207	243	278
71	136	143	150	157	165	172	179	186	183	200	208	215	250	286
72	140	147	154	162	169	177	184	191	199	206	213	221	258	294
73	144	151	159	166	174	182	189	197	204	212	219	227	265	302
74	148	155	163	171	179	186	194	202	210	218	225	233	272	311
75	152	160	168	176	184	192	200	208	216	224	232	240	279	319
76	156	164	172	180	189	197	205	213	221	230	238	246	287	328

Risk of Disease Associated with BMI

Body Mass Number	Definition	Waist size less than or equal to: 40" Men, 35" Women	Waist size that is greater than: 40" in Men, 35" women
18.5 or less	Underweight		
18.5 - 24.9	Normal		
25.0-29.9	Overweight	Increased Risk	High Risk
30.0-34.9	Obese	High Risk	Very High Risk
35.0-39.9	Obese	Very High Risk	Very High Risk
40 or greater	Morbidly Obese	Extremely High Risk	Extremely High Risk

Weight / Body Fat Tracking Chart

Work with your doctor to determine your healthy weight range.
Highlight your healthy weight range on the charts below.

Check One
Body Mass Index
Body Fat Measure

Weight in Lbs. chart

Weight in Lbs.	Date	Date	Date	Date	Date	Date	Date	Date	Date	Date	Date	Date	Date	Date	Date
500															
450															
400															
350															
300															
250															
225															
200															
195															
185															
175															
165															
155															
145															
135															
125															
100															
95															
85															

Body Fat Chart / Body Mass Index

Height in inches																
Choose One		Date	Date	Date	Date	Date	Date	Date	Date	Date	Date	Date	Date	Date	Date
BMI	BF														
35	80%															
30	70%															
29	60%															
28	50%															
27	45%															
26	40%															
25	35%															
24	30%															
23	25%															
22	20%															
21	15%															
20	10%															
19	5%															

Weight / Body Fat Tracking Chart

Work with your doctor to determine your healthy weight range.
Highlight your healthy weight range on the charts below.

Check One
Body Mass Index
Body Fat Measure

Weight in Lbs. chart

Weight in Lbs.	Date	Date	Date	Date	Date	Date	Date	Date	Date	Date	Date	Date	Date	Date	Date
500															
450															
400															
350															
300															
250															
225															
200															
195															
185															
175															
165															
155															
145															
135															
125															
100															
95															
85															

Body Fat Chart / Body Mass Index

Height in inches																
Choose One		Date	Date	Date	Date	Date	Date	Date	Date	Date	Date	Date	Date	Date	Date
BMI	BF															
35	80%															
30	70%															
29	60%															
28	50%															
27	45%															
26	40%															
25	35%															
24	30%															
23	25%															
22	20%															
21	15%															
20	10%															
19	5%															

Weight / Body Fat Tracking Chart

Work with your doctor to determine your healthy weight range.
Highlight your healthy weight range on the charts below.

Check One
Body Mass Index
Body Fat Measure

Weight in Lbs. chart

Weight in Lbs.	Date	Date	Date	Date	Date	Date	Date	Date	Date	Date	Date	Date	Date	Date	Date
500															
450															
400															
350															
300															
250															
225															
200															
195															
185															
175															
165															
155															
145															
135															
125															
100															
95															
85															

Body Fat Chart / Body Mass Index

Height in inches															
Choose One		Date	Date	Date	Date	Date	Date	Date	Date	Date	Date	Date	Date	Date	Date
BMI	BF														
35	80%														
30	70%														
29	60%														
28	50%														
27	45%														
26	40%														
25	35%														
24	30%														
23	25%														
22	20%														
21	15%														
20	10%														
19	5%														

Weight / Body Fat Tracking Chart

Work with your doctor to determine your healthy weight range.
Highlight your healthy weight range on the charts below.

Check One	
	Body Mass Index
	Body Fat Measure

Weight in Lbs. chart

Weight in Lbs.	Date	Date	Date	Date	Date	Date	Date	Date	Date	Date	Date	Date	Date	Date	Date
500															
450															
400															
350															
300															
250															
225															
200															
195															
185															
175															
165															
155															
145															
135															
125															
100															
95															
85															

Body Fat Chart / Body Mass Index

Height in inches																
Choose One		Date	Date	Date	Date	Date	Date	Date	Date	Date	Date	Date	Date	Date	Date
BMI	BF															
35	80%															
30	70%															
29	60%															
28	50%															
27	45%															
26	40%															
25	35%															
24	30%															
23	25%															
22	20%															
21	15%															
20	10%															
19	5%															

Weight/Body Fat Tracking Chart

Weight / Body Fat Tracking Chart

Work with your doctor to determine your healthy weight range.
Highlight your healthy weight range on the charts below.

Check One
Body Mass Index
Body Fat Measure

Weight in Lbs. chart

Weight in Lbs.	Date	Date	Date	Date	Date	Date	Date	Date	Date	Date	Date	Date	Date	Date	Date
500															
450															
400															
350															
300															
250															
225															
200															
195															
185															
175															
165															
155															
145															
135															
125															
100															
95															
85															

Body Fat Chart / Body Mass Index

Height in inches																
Choose One		Date	Date	Date	Date	Date	Date	Date	Date	Date	Date	Date	Date	Date	Date
BMI	BF															
35	80%															
30	70%															
29	60%															
28	50%															
27	45%															
26	40%															
25	35%															
24	30%															
23	25%															
22	20%															
21	15%															
20	10%															
19	5%															

Blood Pressure Tracking Chart

Reading	Date	Date	Date	Date	Date	Date	Date	Date	Date	Date	Date	Date	Date	Date	Date	Date
Systolic																
Danger 180																
High 179																
High 175																
High 170																
High 165																
High 160																
159																
155																
150																
145																
140																
139																
135																
130																
125																
120																
Diastolic																
Danger 110																
High 109																
High 105																
High 100																
99																
95																
90																
89																
85																
80																
75																
70																
65																
60																
55																
50																
45																
40																

Systolic	Diastolic	Potential Follow Up Schedule
130-139	85-89	Elevated/High Normal, recheck in 1 year
140-159	90-99	Stage 1/High Mild, confirm in 2 months
160-179	100-109	Stage 2/High Moderate, evaluate in 1 month
180 or higher	110 or higher	Danger/High Severe, evaluate immediately!!!

Blood Pressure Tracking Chart

Reading	Date	Date	Date	Date	Date	Date	Date	Date	Date	Date	Date	Date	Date	Date	Date	Date
Systolic																
Danger 180																
High 179																
High 175																
High 170																
High 165																
High 160																
159																
155																
150																
145																
140																
139																
135																
130																
125																
120																
Diastolic																
Danger 110																
High 109																
High 105																
High 100																
99																
95																
90																
89																
85																
80																
75																
70																
65																
60																
55																
50																
45																
40																

Systolic	Diastolic	Potential Follow Up Schedule
130-139	85-89	Elevated/High Normal, recheck in 1 year
140-159	90-99	Stage 1/High Mild, confirm in 2 months
160-179	100-109	Stage 2/High Moderate, evaluate in 1 month
180 or higher	110 or higher	Danger/High Severe, evaluate immediately!!!

Blood Pressure Tracking Chart

Reading	Date	Date	Date	Date	Date	Date	Date	Date	Date	Date	Date	Date	Date	Date	Date	Date
Systolic																
Danger 180																
High 179																
High 175																
High 170																
High 165																
High 160																
159																
155																
150																
145																
140																
139																
135																
130																
125																
120																
Diastolic																
Danger 110																
High 109																
High 105																
High 100																
99																
95																
90																
89																
85																
80																
75																
70																
65																
60																
55																
50																
45																
40																

Systolic	Diastolic	Potential Follow Up Schedule
130-139	85-89	Elevated/High Normal, recheck in 1 year
140-159	90-99	Stage 1/High Mild, confirm in 2 months
160-179	100-109	Stage 2/High Moderate, evaluate in 1 month
180 or higher	110 or higher	Danger/High Severe, evaluate immediately!!!

Blood Pressure Tracking Chart

Reading	Date	Date	Date	Date	Date	Date	Date	Date	Date	Date	Date	Date	Date	Date	Date	Date
Systolic																
Danger 180																
High 179																
High 175																
High 170																
High 165																
High 160																
159																
155																
150																
145																
140																
139																
135																
130																
125																
120																
Diastolic																
Danger 110																
High 109																
High 105																
High 100																
99																
95																
90																
89																
85																
80																
75																
70																
65																
60																
55																
50																
45																
40																

Systolic	Diastolic	Potential Follow Up Schedule
130-139	85-89	Elevated/High Normal, recheck in 1 year
140-159	90-99	Stage 1/High Mild, confirm in 2 months
160-179	100-109	Stage 2/High Moderate, evaluate in 1 month
180 or higher	110 or higher	Danger/High Severe, evaluate immediately!!!

Blood Pressure Tracking Chart

Reading	Date	Date	Date	Date	Date	Date	Date	Date	Date	Date	Date	Date	Date	Date	Date	Date
Systolic																
Danger 180																
High 179																
High 175																
High 170																
High 165																
High 160																
159																
155																
150																
145																
140																
139																
135																
130																
125																
120																
Diastolic																
Danger 110																
High 109																
High 105																
High 100																
99																
95																
90																
89																
85																
80																
75																
70																
65																
60																
55																
50																
45																
40																

Systolic	Diastolic	Potential Follow Up Schedule
130-139	85-89	Elevated/High Normal, recheck in 1 year
140-159	90-99	Stage 1/High Mild, confirm in 2 months
160-179	100-109	Stage 2/High Moderate, evaluate in 1 month
180 or higher	110 or higher	Danger/High Severe, evaluate immediately!!!

Cholesterol Tracking Chart

Reading	Date	Date	Date	Date	Date	Date	Date	Date	Date	Date	Date	Date	Date	Date	Date	Date
Overall																
350																
300																
250																
225																
200																
100																
Triglyceride																
500																
450																
400																
300																
250																
200																
150																
100																
50																
LDL																
170																
160																
155																
150																
145																
140																
135																
130																
125																
120																
115																
HDL																
70																
65																
60																
55																
50																
45																
40																
35																
30																

Set up a testing schedule with your doctor to accomplish your overall prevention goals.
If your results are outside the range of normal, modify your testing schedule accordingly.

Cholesterol Tracking Chart

Reading	Date	Date	Date	Date	Date	Date	Date	Date	Date	Date	Date	Date	Date	Date	Date	Date
Overall																
350																
300																
250																
225																
200																
100																
Triglyceride																
500																
450																
400																
300																
250																
200																
150																
100																
50																
LDL																
170																
160																
155																
150																
145																
140																
135																
130																
125																
120																
115																
HDL																
70																
65																
60																
55																
50																
45																
40																
35																
30																

Set up a testing schedule with your doctor to accomplish your overall prevention goals.

If your results are outside the range of normal, modify your testing schedule accordingly.

Cholesterol Tracking Chart

Reading	Date	Date	Date	Date	Date	Date	Date	Date	Date	Date	Date	Date	Date	Date	Date	Date
Overall																
350																
300																
250																
225																
200																
100																
Triglyceride																
500																
450																
400																
300																
250																
200																
150																
100																
50																
LDL																
170																
160																
155																
150																
145																
140																
135																
130																
125																
120																
115																
HDL																
70																
65																
60																
55																
50																
45																
40																
35																
30																

Set up a testing schedule with your doctor to accomplish your overall prevention goals.

If your results are outside the range of normal, modify your testing schedule accordingly.

Cholesterol Tracking Chart

Reading	Date	Date	Date	Date	Date	Date	Date	Date	Date	Date	Date	Date	Date	Date	Date	Date
Overall																
350																
300																
250																
225																
200																
100																
Triglyceride																
500																
450																
400																
300																
250																
200																
150																
100																
50																
LDL																
170																
160																
155																
150																
145																
140																
135																
130																
125																
120																
115																
HDL																
70																
65																
60																
55																
50																
45																
40																
35																
30																

Set up a testing schedule with your doctor to accomplish your overall prevention goals.

If your results are outside the range of normal, modify your testing schedule accordingly.

Cholesterol Tracking Chart

Reading	Date	Date	Date	Date	Date	Date	Date	Date	Date	Date	Date	Date	Date	Date	Date	Date
Overall																
350																
300																
250																
225																
200																
100																
Triglyceride																
500																
450																
400																
300																
250																
200																
150																
100																
50																
LDL																
170																
160																
155																
150																
145																
140																
135																
130																
125																
120																
115																
HDL																
70																
65																
60																
55																
50																
45																
40																
35																
30																

Set up a testing schedule with your doctor to accomplish your overall prevention goals.

If your results are outside the range of normal, modify your testing schedule accordingly.

Tracking Chart For:

Scale	Date	Date	Date	Date	Date	Date	Date	Date	Date	Date	Date	Date	Date	Date	Date	Date

Use this blank tracking chart to monitor readings. Along the left side of the page under Scale mark the range *normal* too *high* for the test you are monitoring. Use one of the *Vital Statistic Tracking Charts* as a guide to make a chart for any vital statistics you are monitoring to maintain or reach your health goals.

Tracking Chart For:

Scale	Date	Date	Date	Date	Date	Date	Date	Date	Date	Date	Date	Date	Date	Date	Date	Date

Use this blank tracking chart to monitor readings. Along the left side of the page under Scale mark the range *normal* too *high* for the test you are monitoring. Use one of the *Vital Statistic Tracking Charts* as a guide to make a chart for any vital statistics you are monitoring to maintain or reach your health goals.

Tracking Chart For:

Scale	Date	Date	Date	Date	Date	Date	Date	Date	Date	Date	Date	Date	Date	Date	Date	Date

Use this blank tracking chart to monitor readings. Along the left side of the page under Scale mark the range *normal* too *high* for the test you are monitoring. Use one of the *Vital Statistic Tracking Charts* as a guide to make a chart for any vital statistics you are monitoring to maintain or reach your health goals.

Tracking Chart For:

Scale	Date	Date	Date	Date	Date	Date	Date	Date	Date	Date	Date	Date	Date	Date	Date	Date

Use this blank tracking chart to monitor readings. Along the left side of the page under Scale mark the range *normal* too *high* for the test you are monitoring. Use one of the *Vital Statistic Tracking Charts* as a guide to make a chart for any vital statistics you are monitoring to maintain or reach your health goals.

Tracking Chart For:

Scale	Date	Date	Date	Date	Date	Date	Date	Date	Date	Date	Date	Date	Date	Date	Date	Date

Use this blank tracking chart to monitor readings. Along the left side of the page under Scale mark the range *normal* too *high* for the test you are monitoring. Use one of the *Vital Statistic Tracking Charts* as a guide to make a chart for any vital statistics you are monitoring to maintain or reach your health goals.

DETECTION

Sometimes we get a series of symptoms, go to the doctor, and are told there is no apparent cause for these symptoms. This is a frustrating situation for both the patient and the doctor. Often a diagnosis cannot be made because not enough information was gathered. When this occurs, you may want to use the *Detection Worksheet*. This worksheet looks similar to the *Office Visit Worksheet*, with some additional places to track the *how's* and *why's* associated with your symptoms, giving you and your doctor a more-detailed map of your condition.

It is important when tracking a health problem to be as detailed as possible. Write down your symptoms and the time that they occur. If your symptoms are pain related, mark the type of pain by placing the letter at the location of your pain using the body figure. Break your symptoms down over time using the *a.m.* and *p.m.* section.

Take your temperature and note the reading and time. If you are tracking your blood pressure at home, take it and note the reading and the time. If you are tracking your blood sugar level at home, take it, and note the reading and the time. Any other home test that you are performing should also be done, and the result and time noted on your *Detection Worksheet*.

Take a minute and write in the answers to these four questions:

•What activity was I doing when this symptom occurred?
Note if you had this symptom after this activity in the past, perhaps mildly, but not worth noting at that time.

•What stress was I under when this symptom occurred?
Stresses can be physical or emotional. Again, make a note if you had this symptom in the past after this kind of stress.

•What foods have I eaten in the last eight hours?

•What medications, vitamins, herbs, or enzymes have I taken in the last two hours?

In the notes and questions section, write in any thoughts you have about your symptoms. When you go back and review your log, you and your doctor may find a common thread in your notes and thoughts that may be useful in making a more accurate diagnosis.

With the *Detection Worksheets,* you and your doctor should have enough information to point you in the right direction. The next 21 pages of your handbook contain *Detection Worksheets*, providing 3 weeks or 21 dates worth of documentation. You could double or triple up the information on each page by writing in different color ink. Or use it to track for a week by writing the date next to each note.

Detection Worksheet

Date:_____   Temperature: <u>AM/</u>_____   PM/_____

Hours of Sleep: _____   Blood Pressure 1:_____/_____   Blood Pressure 2: _____/_____

Blood Sugar 1: _____   Blood Sugar 2: _____

<u>Note in the spaces below the answers to these four questions</u>:

What activity was I doing when these symptoms occurred?

What stress, physical or emotional, was I under when these symptoms occurred?

What foods have I eaten in the last eight hours?

What medications had I taken today?

<u>Pain Type & Location</u>

Write the letter of the type of pain on the figure – or – detail the pain in the systems section:

T=Throbbing, C=Constant, R=Radiating, SQ=Squeezing, P=Pressure, S=Sharp, M=With Movement

Symptoms occurring today: _____

_____

_____

_____

_____

_____

Activities that may have contributed to these symptoms: _____

_____

_____

_____

Foods	Eaten at...	Symptoms improve, get worse, no change?

Medication	Taken at...	Symptoms improve, get worse, no change?

Notes and Questions

Detection Worksheet

Date:_____   Temperature: <u>AM</u>/_____   <u>PM</u>/_____
Hours of Sleep: _____   Blood Pressure 1:____/____ Blood Pressure 2: ____/____
Blood Sugar 1: _____ Blood Sugar 2: _____

<u>Note in the spaces below the answers to these four questions</u>:
What activity was I doing when these symptoms occurred?
What stress, physical or emotional, was I under when these symptoms occurred?
What foods have I eaten in the last eight hours?
What medications had I taken today?

<u>Pain Type & Location</u>
Write the letter of the type of pain on the figure – or – detail the pain in the systems section:
T=Throbbing, C=Constant, R=Radiating, SQ=Squeezing, P=Pressure, S=Sharp, M=With Movement

Symptoms occurring today: _____
_____
_____
_____
_____
_____

Activities that may have contributed to these symptoms: _____
_____
_____
_____

Foods	Eaten at...	Symptoms improve, get worse, no change?

Medication	Taken at...	Symptoms improve, get worse, no change?

Notes and Questions

Detection Worksheet

Date:_____ Temperature: AM/_____ PM/_____

Hours of Sleep: _____ Blood Pressure 1:_____/_____ Blood Pressure 2: _____/_____

Blood Sugar 1: _____ Blood Sugar 2: _____

Note in the spaces below the answers to these four questions:

What activity was I doing when these symptoms occurred?

What stress, physical or emotional, was I under when these symptoms occurred?

What foods have I eaten in the last eight hours?

What medications had I taken today?

Pain Type & Location

Write the letter of the type of pain on the figure – or – detail the pain in the systems section:

T=Throbbing, C=Constant, R=Radiating, SQ=Squeezing, P=Pressure, S=Sharp, M=With Movement

Symptoms occurring today: _____

_____

_____

_____

_____

_____

_____

Activities that may have contributed to these symptoms: _____

_____

_____

_____

Foods	Eaten at...	Symptoms improve, get worse, no change?

Medication	Taken at...	Symptoms improve, get worse, no change?

Notes and Questions

Detection Worksheet

Date:_____   Temperature: <u>AM/</u>_____   PM/_____

Hours of Sleep: _____   Blood Pressure 1:_____/_____ Blood Pressure 2: _____/_____

Blood Sugar 1: _____ Blood Sugar 2: _____

<u>Note in the spaces below the answers to these four questions</u>:

What activity was I doing when these symptoms occurred?

What stress, physical or emotional, was I under when these symptoms occurred?

What foods have I eaten in the last eight hours?

What medications had I taken today?

<u>Pain Type & Location</u>

Write the letter of the type of pain on the figure – or – detail the pain in the systems section:

T=Throbbing, C=Constant, R=Radiating, SQ=Squeezing, P=Pressure, S=Sharp, M=With Movement

Symptoms occurring today: _____

_____

_____

_____

_____

_____

_____

Activities that may have contributed to these symptoms: _____

_____

_____

_____

Foods	Eaten at...	Symptoms improve, get worse, no change?
Medication	Taken at...	Symptoms improve, get worse, no change?
Notes and Questions		

Detection Worksheet

Date:_____   Temperature: AM/_____   PM/_____

Hours of Sleep: _____   Blood Pressure 1:_____/_____ Blood Pressure 2: ____/_____

Blood Sugar 1: _____ Blood Sugar 2: _____

Note in the spaces below the answers to these four questions:

What activity was I doing when these symptoms occurred?

What stress, physical or emotional, was I under when these symptoms occurred?

What foods have I eaten in the last eight hours?

What medications had I taken today?

Pain Type & Location

Write the letter of the type of pain on the figure – or – detail the pain in the systems section:

T=Throbbing, C=Constant, R=Radiating, SQ=Squeezing, P=Pressure, S=Sharp, M=With Movement

Symptoms occurring today: _____

_____

_____

_____

_____

_____

Activities that may have contributed to these symptoms: _____

_____

_____

_____

Foods	Eaten at...	Symptoms improve, get worse, no change?
Medication	Taken at...	Symptoms improve, get worse, no change?
Notes and Questions		

Detection Worksheet

Date:_____   Temperature: <u>AM/</u>_____   <u>PM/</u>_____

Hours of Sleep: _____   Blood Pressure 1:_____/_____ Blood Pressure 2: _____/_____

Blood Sugar 1: _____ Blood Sugar 2: _____

<u>Note in the spaces below the answers to these four questions:</u>

What activity was I doing when these symptoms occurred?

What stress, physical or emotional, was I under when these symptoms occurred?

What foods have I eaten in the last eight hours?

What medications had I taken today?

<u>Pain Type & Location</u>

Write the letter of the type of pain on the figure – or – detail the pain in the systems section:

T=Throbbing, C=Constant, R=Radiating, SQ=Squeezing, P=Pressure, S=Sharp, M=With Movement

Symptoms occurring today: _____

_____

_____

_____

_____

_____

Activities that may have contributed to these symptoms: _____

_____

_____

_____

Foods	Eaten at...	Symptoms improve, get worse, no change?

Medication	Taken at...	Symptoms improve, get worse, no change?

Notes and Questions

Detection Worksheet

Date:_____   Temperature: <u>AM/</u>_____   <u>PM/</u>_____
Hours of Sleep: _____   Blood Pressure 1:_____/_____ Blood Pressure 2: ____/_____
                                   Blood Sugar 1: _____ Blood Sugar 2: _____

<u>Note in the spaces below the answers to these four questions:</u>
What activity was I doing when these symptoms occurred?
What stress, physical or emotional, was I under when these symptoms occurred?
What foods have I eaten in the last eight hours?
What medications had I taken today?

<u>Pain Type & Location</u>
Write the letter of the type of pain on the figure – or – detail the pain in the systems section:
T=Throbbing, C=Constant, R=Radiating, SQ=Squeezing, P=Pressure, S=Sharp, M=With Movement

Symptoms occurring today: _____
_____
_____
_____
_____
_____
_____

Activities that may have contributed to these symptoms: _____
_____
_____
_____

Foods	Eaten at...	Symptoms improve, get worse, no change?
Medication	Taken at...	Symptoms improve, get worse, no change?
Notes and Questions		

Detection Worksheet

Date:_____ Temperature: <u>AM/</u>_____ PM/_____
Hours of Sleep: _____ Blood Pressure 1:____/____ Blood Pressure 2: ___/____
Blood Sugar 1: _____ Blood Sugar 2: _____

<u>Note in the spaces below the answers to these four questions</u>:
What activity was I doing when these symptoms occurred?
What stress, physical or emotional, was I under when these symptoms occurred?
What foods have I eaten in the last eight hours?
What medications had I taken today?

<u>Pain Type & Location</u>
Write the letter of the type of pain on the figure – or – detail the pain in the systems section:
T=Throbbing, C=Constant, R=Radiating, SQ=Squeezing, P=Pressure, S=Sharp, M=With Movement

Symptoms occurring today: _____
_____
_____
_____
_____
_____
_____

Activities that may have contributed to these symptoms: _____
_____
_____
_____

Foods	Eaten at...	Symptoms improve, get worse, no change?

Medication	Taken at...	Symptoms improve, get worse, no change?

Notes and Questions

Detection Worksheet

Date:_____   Temperature: <u>AM/</u>_____ <u>PM/</u>_____

Hours of Sleep: _____   Blood Pressure 1:_____/_____ Blood Pressure 2: _____/_____

Blood Sugar 1: _____ Blood Sugar 2: _____

<u>Note in the spaces below the answers to these four questions:</u>

What activity was I doing when these symptoms occurred?

What stress, physical or emotional, was I under when these symptoms occurred?

What foods have I eaten in the last eight hours?

What medications had I taken today?

<u>Pain Type & Location</u>

Write the letter of the type of pain on the figure – or – detail the pain in the systems section:

T=Throbbing, C=Constant, R=Radiating, SQ=Squeezing, P=Pressure, S=Sharp, M=With Movement

Symptoms occurring today: _____

_____

_____

_____

_____

_____

Activities that may have contributed to these symptoms: _____

_____

_____

_____

Foods	Eaten at...	Symptoms improve, get worse, no change?

Medication	Taken at...	Symptoms improve, get worse, no change?

Notes and Questions

Detection Worksheet

Date:_____   Temperature: <u>AM/</u>_____ <u>PM/</u>_____

Hours of Sleep: _____   Blood Pressure 1:____/_____ Blood Pressure 2: ____/_____

Blood Sugar 1: _____ Blood Sugar 2: _____

<u>Note in the spaces below the answers to these four questions:</u>

What activity was I doing when these symptoms occurred?

What stress, physical or emotional, was I under when these symptoms occurred?

What foods have I eaten in the last eight hours?

What medications had I taken today?

<u>Pain Type & Location</u>

Write the letter of the type of pain on the figure – or – detail the pain in the systems section:

T=Throbbing, C=Constant, R=Radiating, SQ=Squeezing, P=Pressure, S=Sharp, M=With Movement

Symptoms occurring today: _____

_____

_____

_____

_____

_____

_____

Activities that may have contributed to these symptoms: _____

_____

_____

_____

Foods	Eaten at...	Symptoms improve, get worse, no change?
Medication	Taken at...	Symptoms improve, get worse, no change?
Notes and Questions		

Detection Worksheet

Date:_____ Temperature: <u>AM/</u>_____ <u>PM/</u>_____
Hours of Sleep: _____ Blood Pressure 1:_____/_____ Blood Pressure 2: ____/_____
                              Blood Sugar 1: _____ Blood Sugar 2: _____

<u>Note in the spaces below the answers to these four questions:</u>
What activity was I doing when these symptoms occurred?
What stress, physical or emotional, was I under when these symptoms occurred?
What foods have I eaten in the last eight hours?
What medications had I taken today?

<u>Pain Type & Location</u>
Write the letter of the type of pain on the figure – or – detail the pain in the systems section:
T=Throbbing, C=Constant, R=Radiating, SQ=Squeezing, P=Pressure, S=Sharp, M=With Movement

Symptoms occurring today: _____
_____
_____
_____
_____
_____
_____

Activities that may have contributed to these symptoms: _____
_____
_____
_____

Foods	Eaten at...	Symptoms improve, get worse, no change?

Medication	Taken at...	Symptoms improve, get worse, no change?

Notes and Questions

Detection Worksheet

Date:_____   Temperature: <u>AM/</u>_____ <u>PM/</u>_____
Hours of Sleep: _____   Blood Pressure 1:_____/_____ Blood Pressure 2: ____/_____
Blood Sugar 1: _____ Blood Sugar 2: _____

<u>Note in the spaces below the answers to these four questions</u>:
What activity was I doing when these symptoms occurred?
What stress, physical or emotional, was I under when these symptoms occurred?
What foods have I eaten in the last eight hours?
What medications had I taken today?

<u>Pain Type & Location</u>
Write the letter of the type of pain on the figure – or – detail the pain in the systems section:
T=Throbbing, C=Constant, R=Radiating, SQ=Squeezing, P=Pressure, S=Sharp, M=With Movement

Symptoms occurring today: _____
_____
_____
_____
_____
_____
_____

Activities that may have contributed to these symptoms: _____
_____
_____
_____

Foods	Eaten at...	Symptoms improve, get worse, no change?

Medication	Taken at...	Symptoms improve, get worse, no change?

Notes and Questions

Detection Worksheet

Date:_____   Temperature: <u>AM/</u>_____   PM/_____

Hours of Sleep: _____   Blood Pressure 1:_____/_____ Blood Pressure 2: ____/____

Blood Sugar 1: _____ Blood Sugar 2: _____

<u>Note in the spaces below the answers to these four questions</u>:

What activity was I doing when these symptoms occurred?

What stress, physical or emotional, was I under when these symptoms occurred?

What foods have I eaten in the last eight hours?

What medications had I taken today?

<u>Pain Type & Location</u>

Write the letter of the type of pain on the figure – or – detail the pain in the systems section:

T=Throbbing, C=Constant, R=Radiating, SQ=Squeezing, P=Pressure, S=Sharp, M=With Movement

Symptoms occurring today: _____

_____

_____

_____

_____

_____

Activities that may have contributed to these symptoms: _____

_____

_____

_____

Foods	Eaten at...	Symptoms improve, get worse, no change?

Medication	Taken at...	Symptoms improve, get worse, no change?

Notes and Questions

Detection Worksheet

Date:_____   Temperature: <u>AM/</u>_____   <u>PM/</u>_____

Hours of Sleep: _____   Blood Pressure 1:_____/_____   Blood Pressure 2: _____/_____

Blood Sugar 1: _____   Blood Sugar 2: _____

<u>Note in the spaces below the answers to these four questions:</u>

What activity was I doing when these symptoms occurred?

What stress, physical or emotional, was I under when these symptoms occurred?

What foods have I eaten in the last eight hours?

What medications had I taken today?

<u>Pain Type & Location</u>

Write the letter of the type of pain on the figure – or – detail the pain in the systems section:

T=Throbbing, C=Constant, R=Radiating, SQ=Squeezing, P=Pressure, S=Sharp, M=With Movement

Symptoms occurring today: _____

_____

_____

_____

_____

_____

_____

Activities that may have contributed to these symptoms: _____

_____

_____

_____

Foods	Eaten at...	Symptoms improve, get worse, no change?
Medication	Taken at...	Symptoms improve, get worse, no change?
Notes and Questions		

Detection Worksheet

Date:_____   Temperature: <u>AM/</u>_____   PM/_____

Hours of Sleep: _____   Blood Pressure 1:____/____   Blood Pressure 2: ___/____

Blood Sugar 1: _____   Blood Sugar 2: _____

<u>Note in the spaces below the answers to these four questions:</u>

What activity was I doing when these symptoms occurred?

What stress, physical or emotional, was I under when these symptoms occurred?

What foods have I eaten in the last eight hours?

What medications had I taken today?

<u>Pain Type & Location</u>

Write the letter of the type of pain on the figure – or – detail the pain in the systems section:

T=Throbbing, C=Constant, R=Radiating, SQ=Squeezing, P=Pressure, S=Sharp, M=With Movement

Symptoms occurring today: _____

_____

_____

_____

_____

_____

_____

Activities that may have contributed to these symptoms: _____

_____

_____

_____

Foods	Eaten at...	Symptoms improve, get worse, no change?
Medication	Taken at...	Symptoms improve, get worse, no change?
Notes and Questions		

Detection Worksheet

Date:_____   Temperature: <u>AM/</u>_____   PM/_____
Hours of Sleep: _____   Blood Pressure 1:_____/_____ Blood Pressure 2: ____/_____
                                        Blood Sugar 1: _____ Blood Sugar 2: _____

<u>Note in the spaces below the answers to these four questions:</u>
What activity was I doing when these symptoms occurred?
What stress, physical or emotional, was I under when these symptoms occurred?
What foods have I eaten in the last eight hours?
What medications had I taken today?

<u>Pain Type & Location</u>
Write the letter of the type of pain on the figure – or – detail the pain in the systems section:
T=Throbbing, C=Constant, R=Radiating, SQ=Squeezing, P=Pressure, S=Sharp, M=With Movement

Symptoms occurring today: _____
_____
_____
_____
_____
_____

Activities that may have contributed to these symptoms: _____
_____
_____
_____

Foods	Eaten at...	Symptoms improve, get worse, no change?

Medication	Taken at...	Symptoms improve, get worse, no change?

Notes and Questions

Detection Worksheet

Date:_____   Temperature: <u>AM</u>/_____   <u>PM</u>/_____

Hours of Sleep: _____   Blood Pressure 1:____/____   Blood Pressure 2: ____/____

Blood Sugar 1: _____   Blood Sugar 2: _____

<u>Note in the spaces below the answers to these four questions:</u>

What activity was I doing when these symptoms occurred?

What stress, physical or emotional, was I under when these symptoms occurred?

What foods have I eaten in the last eight hours?

What medications had I taken today?

<u>Pain Type & Location</u>

Write the letter of the type of pain on the figure – or – detail the pain in the systems section:

T=Throbbing, C=Constant, R=Radiating, SQ=Squeezing, P=Pressure, S=Sharp, M=With Movement

Symptoms occurring today: _____
_____
_____
_____
_____
_____

Activities that may have contributed to these symptoms: _____
_____
_____
_____

Foods	Eaten at...	Symptoms improve, get worse, no change?

Medication	Taken at...	Symptoms improve, get worse, no change?

Notes and Questions

Detection Worksheet

Date:_____
Hours of Sleep: _____

Temperature: <u>AM</u>/_____ <u>PM</u>/_____
Blood Pressure 1:____/____ Blood Pressure 2: ____/____
Blood Sugar 1: _____ Blood Sugar 2: _____

<u>Note in the spaces below the answers to these four questions:</u>
What activity was I doing when these symptoms occurred?
What stress, physical or emotional, was I under when these symptoms occurred?
What foods have I eaten in the last eight hours?
What medications had I taken today?

<u>Pain Type & Location</u>
Write the letter of the type of pain on the figure – or – detail the pain in the systems section:
T=Throbbing, C=Constant, R=Radiating, SQ=Squeezing, P=Pressure, S=Sharp, M=With Movement

Symptoms occurring today: _____
_____
_____
_____
_____
_____

Activities that may have contributed to these symptoms: _____
_____
_____
_____

Foods	Eaten at...	Symptoms improve, get worse, no change?

Medication	Taken at...	Symptoms improve, get worse, no change?

Notes and Questions

Detection Worksheet

Date:_____ Temperature: AM/_____ PM/_____

Hours of Sleep: _____ Blood Pressure 1:____/____ Blood Pressure 2: ____/____

Blood Sugar 1: _____ Blood Sugar 2: _____

Note in the spaces below the answers to these four questions:

What activity was I doing when these symptoms occurred?

What stress, physical or emotional, was I under when these symptoms occurred?

What foods have I eaten in the last eight hours?

What medications had I taken today?

Pain Type & Location

Write the letter of the type of pain on the figure – or – detail the pain in the systems section:

T=Throbbing, C=Constant, R=Radiating, SQ=Squeezing, P=Pressure, S=Sharp, M=With Movement

Symptoms occurring today: _____

_____

_____

_____

_____

_____

_____

Activities that may have contributed to these symptoms: _____

_____

_____

_____

Foods	Eaten at...	Symptoms improve, get worse, no change?
Medication	Taken at...	Symptoms improve, get worse, no change?
Notes and Questions		

Detection Worksheet

Date:_____   Temperature: <u>AM/</u>_____   PM/_____
Hours of Sleep: _____   Blood Pressure 1:_____/_____   Blood Pressure 2: ____/_____
                                  Blood Sugar 1: _____   Blood Sugar 2: _____

<u>Note in the spaces below the answers to these four questions</u>:
What activity was I doing when these symptoms occurred?
What stress, physical or emotional, was I under when these symptoms occurred?
What foods have I eaten in the last eight hours?
What medications had I taken today?

<u>Pain Type & Location</u>
Write the letter of the type of pain on the figure – or – detail the pain in the systems section:
T=Throbbing, C=Constant, R=Radiating, SQ=Squeezing, P=Pressure, S=Sharp, M=With Movement

Symptoms occurring today: _____
_____
_____
_____
_____
_____
_____

Activities that may have contributed to these symptoms: _____
_____
_____
_____

Foods	Eaten at...	Symptoms improve, get worse, no change?

Medication	Taken at...	Symptoms improve, get worse, no change?

Notes and Questions

Detection Worksheet

Date:_____   Temperature: <u>AM/</u>_____   <u>PM/</u>_____

Hours of Sleep: _____   Blood Pressure 1:_____/_____ Blood Pressure 2: ____/_____

Blood Sugar 1: _____ Blood Sugar 2: _____

<u>Note in the spaces below the answers to these four questions:</u>

What activity was I doing when these symptoms occurred?

What stress, physical or emotional, was I under when these symptoms occurred?

What foods have I eaten in the last eight hours?

What medications had I taken today?

<u>Pain Type & Location</u>

Write the letter of the type of pain on the figure – or – detail the pain in the systems section:

T=Throbbing, C=Constant, R=Radiating, SQ=Squeezing, P=Pressure, S=Sharp, M=With Movement

Symptoms occurring today: _____

_____

_____

_____

_____

_____

Activities that may have contributed to these symptoms: _____

_____

_____

_____

Foods	Eaten at...	Symptoms improve, get worse, no change?
Medication	Taken at...	Symptoms improve, get worse, no change?
Notes and Questions		

NOTES:

CHRONIC ILLNESS

The *Detection Worksheet* can also be used for those with a chronic illness. When dealing with a chronic illness, monitoring your symptoms can lead to keeping many potential problems under control. Catching small changes before they become big changes will give you and your healthcare provider time to modify your treatment strategy.

It is important to be as detailed as possible when writing down your symptoms. If you are having pain with your chronic illness, I recommend creating a *Pain-tracking Chart* with one of the blank graph sheets. Answer the four questions, or change them to questions that are more appropriate for your chronic illness. Note the foods, medications and vitamins that you have been taking and any side effects that you might be experiencing.

Finally, use the *Blood Pressure Tracking Chart, Weight Chart, Cholesterol Tracking Chart, Blood Sugar Tracking Chart,* or create a chart with your doctor specifically designed to track your chronic illness symptoms.

For some with chronic illness tracking multiple symptoms or test readings on a chart may be ideal, for others just using a separate daily calendar in the computer on your phone or just a paper calendar to jot down the readings might be easier. Just remember to bring that information with you to your doctor appointments or review them before your visit and note any changes to discuss with your doctor on your *Office Visit Worksheet*.

What you are looking for are changes in your symptoms or any new symptoms so you can put measures into place to deal with them as soon as you can detect them.

With this information, you and your healthcare provider can keep your chronic illness closely monitored with accurate historical health status charting instead of just a snapshot and a having to remember how you felt or what your test readings where on a given day. Giving you more control over your health, general well-being and ultimately, your life.

ESCALATION OF A PROBLEM

There may be times when you and your insurance provider, or you and your healthcare provider do not see eye to eye. No matter how uncomfortable it is to argue with an insurance bureaucrat or a medical doctor, your good health is worth the discomfort. Getting the care you need is your right, but only if you exercise that right.

The *Escalation Log* on the following pages is a tool you can use to maintain the written information you need to move toward the resolution of any differences you and your healthcare providers may have. Not all battles with your healthcare provider can be won, but without good documentation your fight may be much more difficult. In today's cost-containment focused world, good documentation may put you in a much stronger position to get what you want or need. Knowing the order and timing that conversations occur along with the topic can also keep you from getting into one of those "infinite loop" situations and instead continue to move forward to a successful outcome.

If you are having difficulty receiving the approval you and your doctor would like, you can try and take it a step further with documented back-up information. If you need a particular test or treatment that has been refused by your insurance provider, contact the organization that recommends that test for your age or family health history, obtain copies of the necessary literature, get written details about that treatment from a second doctor or from health organizations that have the documentation to support your request and include them with your next request. If you are prepared and have done your homework, the more likely you are to achieve a positive outcome. Unfortunately, we can't always count on our healthcare provider to do all the leg work; take control of as much as you can to make sure you don't fall thru the cracks of your doctor's super busy schedule. Use your doctor to navigate thru to the result you both want.

If you are passed from doctor to doctor and getting different or conflicting information, noting down who said what in chronological order as you move thru the process can be more useful than trying to remember. Often, we just assume our doctors all discussing our personal health situation and are all on the same page. There is a chance your doctors are not talking to each other or referencing each other's notes about you. Which leads me to this story.

One of my work colleagues Mom was having terrible pain in her back. She was passed from doctor to doctor having no true diagnosis and continued to be in terrible pain. The doctors who saw her all had different guesses as to what it was, none of them seemed serious. Yet my friend kept pressing because her Mom was not getting any relief. Frustrated, my friend pushed aggressively for the right tests to be done and they found Osteomyelitis: an infection in the bone in her upper spine and a subsequent abscess that would need to be removed surgically. The doctors were going to send her home with pain medication, without knowing what was the cause of the pain. If the abscess had gone untreated, eventually it would have gotten so big it could have paralyzed her for life. My friend had been pressing the doctors starting on a Friday morning to get them to take this pain seriously, finally on the following Tuesday they had the real answer and surgery was done that Thursday. She will have a long recovery of over three months, but she will be walking and continue to be independent and enjoy her life.

Not everyone is as organized as my friend. The *Escalation Log* may help you keep track of the details of your dilemma, as well as with whom you spoke, and the promises made to you. Remember, you are not complaining!

You have a right to be involved in your treatments, testing and overall health strategies.

Escalation Log

Date:	Attending Doctor:
	Attending Nurse:
	Others who can give details:

Details of Request or Complaint:

Phone:	Date:	Time:	Contact:

Were the details of your complaint relayed to this person?   Yes / No

Resolution Desired:

Were you referred to someone else?	Who?	Phone:

What is their next action?

What is your next action?

Phone:	Date:	Time:	Contact:

Were the details of your complaint relayed to this person?   Yes / No

Resolution Desired:

Were you referred to someone else?	Who?	Phone:

What is their next action?

What is your next action?

*Additional log listing on the next page

Continuing log entries for unresolved complaint.

Phone:	Date:	Time:	Contact:
Were the details of your complaint relayed to this person? Yes / No			
Resolution Desired:			

Were you referred to someone else?	Who?	Phone:
What is their next action?		

What is your next action?

Phone:	Date:	Time:	Contact:
Were the details of your complaint relayed to this person? Yes / No			
Resolution Desired:			

Were you referred to someone else?	Who?	Phone:
What is their next action?		

What is your next action?

Phone:	Date:	Time:	Contact:
Were the details of your complaint relayed to this person? Yes / No			
Resolution Desired:			

Were you referred to someone else?	Who?	Phone:
What is their next action?		

What is your next action?

If you have already filled this in, use it as a guide to write notes on a separate piece of paper.
I hope you never have to fill this out and all your healthcare interactions go smoothly.

SERIOUS ILLNESS

One of the more frightening situations a person can experience is being confronted with a diagnosis of a serious illness. Often this type of diagnosis can leave you speechless and in shock. Scared and confused, you may not get all the information you need to make the best decisions regarding your treatment. You know that you should be asking questions, they just don't make it to your lips. When it comes to serious illness, ignorance is not bliss. Quite the opposite, the *more* you know the stronger you become.

In creating the worksheets for *Serious Illness, Family Member,* and *Caregiver,* it is my goal to provide tools for you to gain more control at this critical time. The *Serious Illness Worksheet* is one I hope you never have to use; however, *The Smart Patient's Healthcare Handbook* is designed to enable you to be more prepared in the event this situation does arise.

If your doctor announces to you that you are seriously ill, turn your handbook to Page 134, and ask the questions provided. These are not all the questions you will ever have, but they are the starting point.

These basic questions will help you:
•   Absorb your situation
•   Prompt additional questions more specific to your illness
•   Request detailed information from your doctor.

Space is provided for you and your doctor to review treatment options and timetables for decision-making. After your appointment, I encourage you to highlight any questions your doctor could not answer and write down any questions you and your family may have. You can ask these additional questions during your next visit or phone your doctor during their office hours. You also want to ask these same questions during your second-opinion appointment. Several copies of the *Serious Illness Worksheets* are in your handbook for that purpose.

In addition to a brief reference to treatment options on the *Serious Illness Worksheets, Treatment Option Worksheets* are provided as stand-alone documents. Use them to note detailed information about each treatment option as you review them with your doctor, and as you collect additional information on that particular treatment.

If your friends or family will be involved in your treatment, fill in the *Family Member Worksheet* for them to use. Once you have filled in the top section of the *Family Member Worksheet,* make as many copies of the worksheet as you will need to hand out, then personalize each one in the note section at the bottom of the page. The *Family Member Worksheet* will provide the information your friends and family members will need to help you, in an easy-to-understand format.

Giving each friend or family member a clear picture of your situation can help all of you feel more in control during this stress-filled time. The *Family Member Worksheet* will also give you a quiet way to ask for help during your treatment. Many people find asking for help the hardest part of their road back to wellness.

Accept the help; it will ease your stress so you can concentrate on getting well.

Serious Illness Worksheet

Date:_____ Diagnosis (proper spelling):_____

Explanation of this diagnosis:_(if your diagnosis is cancer additional questions are on page 2)_ _____

_____

_____

Does it go by any other names?_____

Where can I find out more about this diagnosis?_____

_____

Are there any other conditions this could be mistaken for?_____

_____

Is this condition contagious or hereditary?_____

Who should I notify to also be tested?_____

Who are the specialists I will be referred to?_____

_____

Will I need surgery? _(see page 2 for more surgery questions)_ _____

What are the top 3 treatment options for me? _(use treatment options worksheet for details)_ ____

_____

_____

Which treatment do you recommend and why?_____

_____

_____

What is the procedure for getting a second opinion? _____

_____

_____

How soon should I make a treatment selection?_____

_____

Can I make dietary changes that will improve my prognosis?_____

_____

What alternative therapies are you aware of that could improve my prognosis?_ _Circle all that should be investigated_

Acupressure   Chelation   Chiropractic   Massage/type:_____

Meditation   Vitamin   Herbal   Other: _____

_____

May I have a copy of the test results you reviewed to make this diagnosis?

I would like to continue to receive copies of all testing done from this time forward.

What are your office hours in case I have further questions? _____

**If you decide to get a second opinion, schedule that as soon as possible. If you are referred to a specialist schedule that as soon as possible. Procrastination and denial steal your power. Don't delay. Keep moving forward.**

Serious Illness Worksheet (continued)

If your diagnosis is cancer. Specify what type:_____

What stage?_____ What does that mean for this type of cancer? _____

_____

Will I need to be hospitalized?_____ If so for how long?_____

Are there clinical trials for my condition?_____

If yes, at what point do we investigate those?_____

_____

What are the risks in treating this type of cancer?_____

_____

_____

_____

If you need surgery

How long will I have to stay in the hospital after surgery?_____

What preparations do I need to make before surgery? *(Mentally, Physically & Nutritionally)*_____

_____

_____

_____

What changes will I need to make after surgery? *(Physically, Nutritionally & Lifestyle)*_____

_____

_____

_____

Will I be able to continue my normal activities after surgery?_____When?_____

What are the chances my illness will return?_____

How will you determine this treatment/surgery is successful?_____

_____

Notes and Additional Information:_____

_____

_____

_____

_____

_____

_____

_____

_____

_____

_____

_____

Treatment Options Worksheet

Suggest you bring a separate notebook to write any additional questions, thoughts, etc...

Name of Treatment:_____

Other names for this treatment?_____

Will I be seeing a doctor other than you to receive this treatment?_____

(if yes) Doctor's name(s):_____

_____

Will this treatment require hospitalization?_____How long?_____

How should I expect to feel during this therapy?_____

In detail, describe this treatment:_____

_____

_____

_____

_____

What are the chances this treatment will be successful?_____

What are the risks of this treatment?_____

_____

What are the side effects I should expect with this treatment?_____

_____

_____

_____

What can I do to lessen the expected side effects?_____

_____

_____

_____

Will there be any long-term effects from this treatment?_____

_____

When would this treatment begin and end?_____

When can I return to normal activity?_____

What drugs would I be taking and side effects of each?_____

_____

_____

_____

_____

What signs will show my condition is improving with this treatment?_____

_____

_____

_____

What signs will show my condition is worsening?_____

_____

_____

How soon must a decision be made?_____

Who will be my primary caregiver during this treatment?_____

Treatment Options Worksheet

Suggest you bring a separate notebook to write any additional questions, thoughts, etc...

Name of Treatment:_____

Other names for this treatment?_____

Will I be seeing a doctor other than you to receive this treatment?_____

(if yes) Doctor's name(s):_____

_____

Will this treatment require hospitalization?_____How long?_____

How should I expect to feel during this therapy?_____

In detail, describe this treatment:_____

_____

_____

_____

_____

What are the chances this treatment will be successful?_____

What are the risks of this treatment?_____

_____

What are the side effects I should expect with this treatment?_____

_____

_____

_____

What can I do to lessen the expected side effects?_____

_____

_____

_____

Will there be any long-term effects from this treatment?_____

_____

When would this treatment begin and end?_____

When can I return to normal activity?_____

What drugs would I be taking and side effects of each?_____

_____

_____

_____

What signs will show my condition is improving with this treatment?_____

_____

_____

_____

What signs will show my condition is worsening?_____

_____

_____

How soon must a decision be made?_____

Who will be my primary caregiver during this treatment?_____

Treatment Options Worksheet

Suggest you bring a separate notebook to write any additional questions, thoughts, etc...

Name of Treatment:_____

Other names for this treatment?_____

Will I be seeing a doctor other than you to receive this treatment?_____

(if yes) Doctor's name(s):_____

_____

Will this treatment require hospitalization?_____How long?_____

How should I expect to feel during this therapy?_____

In detail, describe this treatment:_____

_____

_____

_____

_____

What are the chances this treatment will be successful?_____

What are the risks of this treatment?_____

_____

What are the side effects I should expect with this treatment?_____

_____

_____

_____

What can I do to lessen the expected side effects?_____

_____

_____

_____

Will there be any long-term effects from this treatment?_____

_____

When would this treatment begin and end?_____

When can I return to normal activity?_____

What drugs would I be taking and side effects of each?_____

_____

_____

_____

What signs will show my condition is improving with this treatment?_____

_____

_____

What signs will show my condition is worsening?_____

_____

_____

How soon must a decision be made?_____

Who will be my primary caregiver during this treatment?_____

Family Members & Friends Worksheet

This is my illness:_____Briefly, this means:_____
_____
_____
You can gather more information here:_____

I have Crossed out all that do not apply below
This illness in **NOT** contagious: This illness is **NOT** hereditary:
This illness is contagious – **Get Tested**
This illness may be hereditary – **Get Tested or add to your future testing schedule**

Dietary guidelines that I should be following are:_____
_____
_____
_____

Activities that should be encouraged are:_____
_____
_____
_____

Activities that should be restricted are:_____
_____
_____
_____

Medications that I will be taking are:_____
_____
_____
_____
_____

Possible side effects to watch for are:_____
_____
_____
_____

Prognosis under my current treatment is:_____
_____
_____
_____

Things I may need help with during my treatment & recovery, can you volunteer some time to help?
Shopping   Driving to/from appointments   Sit with me after a treatment to monitor
Cooking   Child Care   if I am not supposed to be on my own
Light Housework   Pet Care

Note:_____
_____
_____
_____

Serious Illness Worksheet

Date:_____   Diagnosis (proper spelling):_____

Explanation of this diagnosis:_(if your diagnosis is cancer additional questions are on page 2)_____

_____

_____

Does it go by any other names?_____

Where can I find out more about this diagnosis?_____

_____

Are there any other conditions this could be mistaken for?_____

_____

Is this condition contagious or hereditary?_____

Who should I notify to also be tested?_____

Who are the specialists I will be referred to?_____

_____

Will I need surgery? _(see page 2 for more surgery questions)_____

What are the top 3 treatment options for me? _(use treatment options worksheet for details)_____

_____

_____

Which treatment do you recommend and why?_____

_____

_____

What is the procedure for getting a second opinion? _____

_____

_____

How soon should I make a treatment selection?_____

_____

Can I make dietary changes that will improve my prognosis?_____

_____

What alternative therapies are you aware of that could improve my prognosis? _Circle all that should be investigated_

Acupressure   Chelation   Chiropractic   Massage/type:_____

Meditation   Vitamin   Herbal   Other: _____

_____

_____

May I have a copy of the test results you reviewed to make this diagnosis?

I would like to continue to receive copies of all testing done from this time forward.

What are your office hours in case I have further questions? _____

If you decide to get a second opinion, schedule that as soon as possible. If you are referred to a specialist schedule that as soon as possible. Procrastination and denial steal your power. Don't delay. Keep moving forward.

Serious Illness Worksheet (continued)

If your diagnosis is cancer. Specify what type:_____

What stage?_____ What does that mean for this type of cancer? _____

_____

Will I need to be hospitalized?_____ If so for how long?_____

Are there clinical trials for my condition?_____

If yes, at what point do we investigate those?_____

_____

What are the risks in treating this type of cancer?_____

_____

_____

_____

If you need surgery

How long will I have to stay in the hospital after surgery?_____

What preparations do I need to make before surgery? *(Mentally, Physically & Nutritionally)*

_____

_____

_____

What changes will I need to make after surgery? *(Physically, Nutritionally & Lifestyle)*

_____

_____

_____

Will I be able to continue my normal activities after surgery?_____When?_____

What are the chances my illness will return?_____

How will you determine this treatment/surgery is successful?_____

_____

Notes and Additional Information:_____

_____

_____

_____

_____

_____

_____

_____

_____

_____

_____

_____

Treatment Options Worksheet

Suggest you bring a separate notebook to write any additional questions, thoughts, etc...

Name of Treatment:_____

Other names for this treatment?_____

Will I be seeing a doctor other than you to receive this treatment?_____

(if yes) Doctor's name(s):_____

_____

Will this treatment require hospitalization?_____How long?_____

How should I expect to feel during this therapy?_____

In detail, describe this treatment:_____

_____

_____

_____

_____

What are the chances this treatment will be successful?_____

What are the risks of this treatment?_____

_____

What are the side effects I should expect with this treatment?_____

_____

_____

What can I do to lessen the expected side effects?_____

_____

_____

Will there be any long-term effects from this treatment?_____

_____

When would this treatment begin and end?_____

When can I return to normal activity?_____

What drugs would I be taking and side effects of each?_____

_____

_____

_____

What signs will show my condition is improving with this treatment?_____

_____

_____

What signs will show my condition is worsening?_____

_____

_____

How soon must a decision be made?_____

Who will be my primary caregiver during this treatment?_____

Treatment Options Worksheet

Suggest you bring a separate notebook to write any additional questions, thoughts, etc...

Name of Treatment:_____

Other names for this treatment?_____

Will I be seeing a doctor other than you to receive this treatment?_____

(if yes) Doctor's name(s):_____

_____

Will this treatment require hospitalization?_____How long?_____

How should I expect to feel during this therapy?_____

In detail, describe this treatment:_____

_____

_____

_____

_____

What are the chances this treatment will be successful?_____

What are the risks of this treatment?_____

_____

What are the side effects I should expect with this treatment?_____

_____

_____

_____

What can I do to lessen the expected side effects?_____

_____

_____

_____

Will there be any long-term effects from this treatment?_____

_____

When would this treatment begin and end?_____

When can I return to normal activity?_____

What drugs would I be taking and side effects of each?_____

_____

_____

_____

_____

What signs will show my condition is improving with this treatment?_____

_____

_____

What signs will show my condition is worsening?_____

_____

_____

How soon must a decision be made?_____

Who will be my primary caregiver during this treatment?_____

Treatment Options Worksheet

Suggest you bring a separate notebook to write any additional questions, thoughts, etc...

Name of Treatment:_____

Other names for this treatment?_____

Will I be seeing a doctor other than you to receive this treatment?_____

(if yes) Doctor's name(s):_____
_____

Will this treatment require hospitalization?_____How long?_____

How should I expect to feel during this therapy?_____

In detail, describe this treatment:_____
_____
_____
_____
_____

What are the chances this treatment will be successful?_____

What are the risks of this treatment?_____
_____

What are the side effects I should expect with this treatment?_____
_____
_____
_____

What can I do to lessen the expected side effects?_____
_____
_____
_____

Will there be any long-term effects from this treatment?_____
_____

When would this treatment begin and end?_____

When can I return to normal activity?_____

What drugs would I be taking and side effects of each?_____
_____
_____
_____

What signs will show my condition is improving with this treatment?_____
_____
_____

What signs will show my condition is worsening?_____
_____
_____

How soon must a decision be made?_____

Who will be my primary caregiver during this treatment?_____

Family Members & Friends Worksheet

This is my illness:_____Briefly, this means:_____
_____
_____

You can gather more information here:_____

I have Crossed out all that do not apply below

This illness in **NOT** contagious: This illness is **NOT** hereditary:

This illness is contagious – **Get Tested**

This illness may be hereditary – **Get Tested or add to your future testing schedule**

Dietary guidelines that I should be following are:_____
_____
_____
_____

Activities that should be encouraged are:_____
_____
_____
_____

Activities that should be restricted are:_____
_____
_____
_____

Medications that I will be taking are:_____
_____
_____
_____

Possible side effects to watch for are:_____
_____
_____
_____

Prognosis under my current treatment is:_____
_____
_____
_____

Things I may need help with during my treatment & recovery, can you volunteer some time to help?

Shopping   Driving to/from appointments   Sit with me after a treatment to monitor
Cooking   Child Care   if I am not supposed to be on my own
Light Housework   Pet Care

Note:_____
_____
_____
_____

CAREGIVER

The *Caregiver Worksheets* are here to be used if your illness requires in-home care. These worksheets are designed for a family member or friend that is providing care; not everyone requires or can afford a hired professional caregiver. They can also be filled out and used to give a hired professional caregiver their starting guidelines.

The first worksheet looks similar to the *Family Member Worksheet*. The caregiver will have additional responsibilities for dietary guidelines, progression of treatment, appointment schedules, physical therapy tracking, and contact information. In addition to calendar/appointment diary, these worksheets can be filled out with the help of your doctor or your doctor's assistant.

You may want to provide your caregiver with copies of your *Prescription Log, Vital Statistic Tracking Charts*, and blank *Detection Worksheets*. Your caregiver can help keep those logs up to date for you and monitor your progress as you get better. I recommend that you make photocopies of all the worksheets your caregiver will need. Have your caregiver create a binder to use during your illness. Your caregiver should use the worksheets listed above, and any additional worksheets in the handbook that can be used to provide you with the best documentation to supervise your speedy recovery.

You may want your caregiver to keep an appointment diary. That diary can also be used to jot down additional information that can be shown to the doctor as a daily log. There are many "day at a glance" type notebooks on the market that would probably work the best, providing lots of room to write.

As with all the worksheets, you should add and delete information as it pertains to your individual situation. These worksheets are just to get you started. As questions come up, include them. As different conditions need to be tracked, monitor them with an existing worksheet, or create a graph with one of the blank tracking charts.

Adjust your worksheets to your individual needs.
Modify any calendar or notebook to your individual needs.

Caregiver Worksheet

Overview

Illness:_____Symptoms:_____
_____

Sources for more information about this condition can be found here:_____
_____

Dietary guidelines that I should be following are: *(see menu worksheet for more details)*___
_____
_____

Activities that should be encouraged are:_____
_____
_____

Activities that should be restricted are:_____
_____
_____

Medications and possible side effects list: *(list here or use prescription log)*_____
_____
_____
_____
_____

Current treatment overview:_____
_____

Prognosis with current treatment:_____
Signs that show improvement:_____
Signs that show regression:_____
Report changes in condition to the following people below –primary or highlighted.

List of important personal contacts:
My Doctor:_____Phone:_____
Pharmacy:_____Phone:_____
Primary Family Contact:_____Phone:_____
_____Phone:_____
_____Phone:_____
_____Phone:_____
_____Phone:_____
_____Phone:_____
_____Phone:_____
_____Phone:_____
_____Phone:_____

Caregiver Worksheet

Dietary Guide and Menu Planner

Approved Foods I Like	Foods to Avoid (even if I like them)

My Favorite Meals

Breakfasts:_____

Lunches:_____

Dinners:_____

Snacks:_____

Caregiver Prescription Log

Medication:_____ For:_____ | P V H A E HO |

Dosage Info:_____ Side Effects:_____

_____

Start Date:_____ Stop Date:_____

Result?_____

Medication:_____ For:_____ | P V H A E HO |

Dosage Info:_____ Side Effects:_____

_____

Start Date:_____ Stop Date:_____

Result?_____

Medication:_____ For:_____ | P V H A E HO |

Dosage Info:_____ Side Effects:_____

_____

Start Date:_____ Stop Date:_____

Result?_____

Medication:_____ For:_____ | P V H A E HO |

Dosage Info:_____ Side Effects:_____

_____

Start Date:_____ Stop Date:_____

Result?_____

Medication:_____ For:_____ | P V H A E HO |

Dosage Info:_____ Side Effects:_____

_____

Start Date:_____ Stop Date:_____

Result?_____

| P=Prescription, V=Vitamin, H=Herb, A=Amino Acid, E=Enzyme, HO=Homeopathic Remedy |

CONCLUSION

It is common knowledge that an ounce of prevention is worth a pound of cure. In relation to the cost of healthcare, an ounce of prevention can be far less expensive than a pound of cure as well. In relation to your quality of life, an ounce of prevention can be a lifetime of feeling great. Instead of spending weeks, maybe years not feeling well, my hope is that these worksheets can assist you and your doctor in targeting conditions as early as possible. When you bring complete information to your physician, along with the proper questions, you create a situation where excellent medicine can be practiced.

The time doctors can spend with their patient's decreases as the pressure for higher profits and bureaucratic red tape increases. If you want to avoid becoming a medical commodity, then you must take control and actively participate in your own healthcare. This workbook is just one tool in your arsenal to protect your quality of life. You now have a record of your health that is under your control no matter which doctor you see or which health insurance carrier you have.

I don't have all the questions you will ever need to ask your doctors tucked into these few pages. My wish for you is that you use these worksheets to capacity. Take a few extra minutes asking questions when you don't understand the situation. Write in the margins if there is no more space on the page. Take notes on separate pieces of paper if you must. Have the doctor's office staffs provide copies of any information you need.

Ask questions, ask questions, ask questions…

Write down the answers

Because you can never know enough about

You!

www.ingramcontent.com/pod-product-compliance
Lightning Source LLC
Chambersburg PA
CBHW080832220526
45467CB00008B/2260